THE SIMPLE ESSENTIAL OILS GUIDE FOR BEGINNERS

The #1 Natural Resource for Weight Loss, Anti-Aging, Natural Cures and Healthy Lifestyles

JOY LOUIS

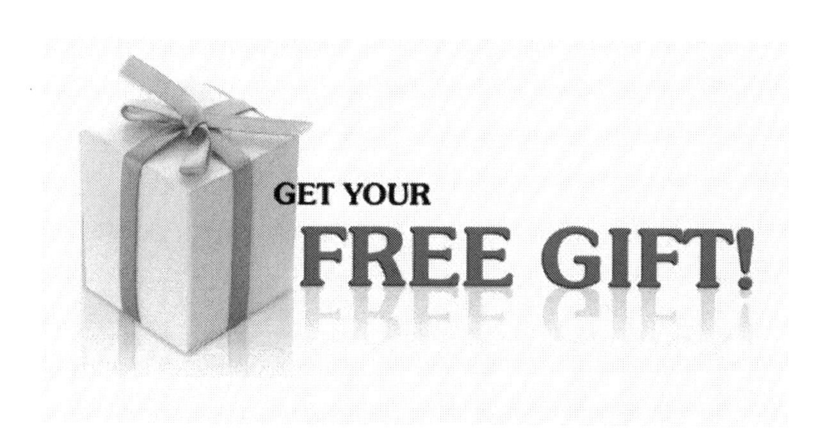

WAIT! BEFORE YOU CONTINUE – DO YOU LIKE FREE BOOKS?

My **FREE Gift** to You!! As a way to say **Thank You** for downloading my book, I'd like to offer you more **FREE BOOKS!** Each time we release a NEW book, we offer it first to a small number of people as a test–drive. Because of your commitment here in downloading my book, I'd love for you to be a part of this group. You can join easily here→ **http://joylouisbooks.com/**

Do You Enjoy **FREE BOOKS**? Do you like books that are Life Changing, Inspirational, Motivational and Informative? We **LOVE** sharing **FREE BOOKS** with people like you. It's easy to join just by clicking here→ **http://joylouisbooks.com/**

BEFORE CONTINUING – FREE BOOKS!

From the Author Joy Louis

Contents

From Author Joy Louis:

I'm so very excited and honored that you've picked up this book and want to learn more about essential oils!

Before you read on and really dive into the book let me introduce myself…

My name is Joy, and I'm an all Natural-Organic-Homemade "Everything" Person. In other words: I have a natural solution for pretty much everything in my life!

My "all natural" way of living started a few years back when I was sick and tired of being sick, FAT and tired. I was eating pretty healthy (or so I thought): I ate peanut butter jelly sandwiches for lunch every day, snacked on cereal protein bars in between meals (these are healthy, right?) and drank Diet Coke (because isn't Diet Coke better than sugar? No calories versus a mother lode of sugar that would go straight to my butt. I'll take the "no sugar" please and thank you). However, despite living my so-called "healthy" lifestyle, I kept gaining weight, and lost all energy and motivation to do anything; I even started to dread taking my dearest Pretzel (my sweet dog of 7 years) out for her daily walk around the neighborhood!

That's when I knew I'd had enough. I decided to start searching for a better way; a way that has now proven to give me more energy than I ever imagined possible and also helped me lose 45 pounds of stubborn body fat in the process. I made a drastic change, 180-degree turn in all my habits.

So here it is. My so called "secret, hidden formula" I used to get to where I am today is: I went ALL NATURAL. Not a very sexy answer, is it? Well I have to tell you, a lot of times we complicate things way too much when looking for an answer. More often than not the solution to our problems is very simple. However... simple doesn't mean it's easy - far from it!

As for me, I don't know how I gathered the willpower to do this, but somehow I managed to throw out all of my garbage foods (i.e cereal bars, cookies, chips and so on) and replaced them with organic, GMO-free vegetables, fruits and lean meats all within **one** day. I completely went cold turkey: I stopped using all of the popular soaps and lotions out there that are FILLED with toxins, and instead I made my own, or found other safe brands and options. A short time after my big lifestyle change I learned about essential oils, and soon they became a necessity in my every day life. They are such an important part of my life and have helped me so much that I have now written a book about them. The world needs to know about these oils, their healing properties and the overall well-being of the people who use them!

As for myself, I use them in almost everything. They're my go-to problem solver, my all-natural medicine cabinet. No more artificial pain killers or medicine with a hundred possible side effects. Essential oils keep my food cravings in check, clear out my sinuses when feel a cold coming on, straighten out the wrinkles and lines coming on in my face, and uplifts my mood the days I feel anxious. For the first time in my life, I can finally say I feel 100% present and alive! I have started to love my body and I have found a true passion in helping others, hence why I decided to write this book. I truly hope you find this book helpful, and please let me know if you have any questions about any of the content.

With much love,

Joy Louis

Introduction

I want to thank you and congratulate you for downloading the book, "*Essential Oils for Beginners.*"

This book contains proven steps and strategies on how to use and understand Eessential Ooils.

Aromatherapy and the use of essential oils is gaining in popularity and is considered to be one of the leading complementary healthcare approaches. Rapid developments in stress-related diseases and aromatic medicine have expanded to create an entirely new study of how the body responds to stimuli and smells.

Essential oils are used in aromatherapy and other traditional and ancient medicinal systems. There are numerous health benefits of essential oils and they are being studied by the medical and scientific communities. Essential oils are complementary treatments for a variety of diseases including cancer, HIV, asthma, bronchitis, heart attacks, strokes, and many more.

There are more than 100 essential oils, and each oil has its own health benefits. Essential oils blend well with each other to form a vast natural medicine cabinet of aromatic combinations. Massage therapy, nursing, esthetics, psychology and hospice and nursing home care professionals are always seeking ways to watch out for the well-being and health of their charges.

There are many essential oils being studied for their use in healthcare, personal care and home care. Massage, inhalation, compresses and alternative healing, as well as personal care products and cleaning creations are only a few of the ways essential oils help make your life easier.

There is a need to understand what essential oils are and what they can do. Essential oils are very light and not greasy. They evaporate quickly and are absorbed into the skin quickly. Essential oils come from the distillation of plant parts including the bark, roots, leaves and flowers. The beauty of essential oils is their fragrance and volatility. Essential oils are used in aromatherapy, alternative medicine pharmaceuticals, cosmetics, perfumery, and many other applications. Essential oils are nature's way of providing a healthy and happy life.

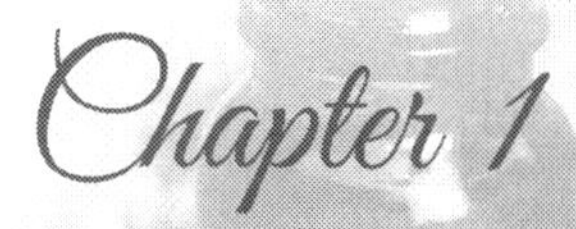

What are Essential Oils?

The term "essential oil" is a contraction of the original "quintessential oil." This stems from the Aristotelian idea that matter is composed of four elements, namely, fire, air, earth, and water. The fifth element, or quintessence, was then considered to be spirit or life force.

History

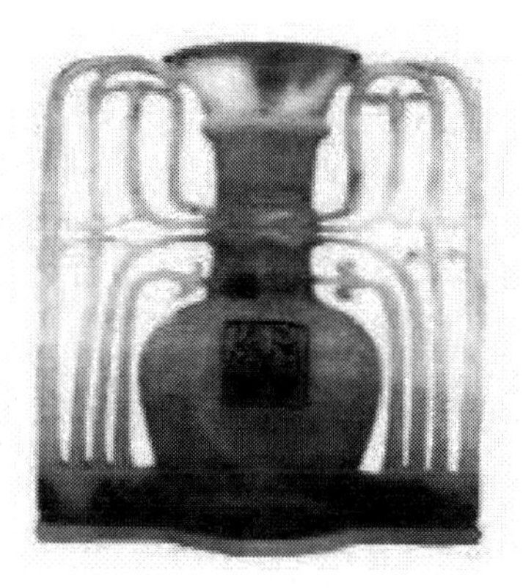

Essential oils are mankind's first medicines. Egyptian Hieroglyphics found on tomb walls prove that essential oils were used in the embalming process, in healing ceremonies, religion, cosmetics and for other medicinal purposes. Recipes for these oils and their uses were first found on the Ebers Papyrus, a medical scroll over 870 feet long. The scroll had over 800 herbal preparations, essential oil recipes and remedies. Other ancient scrolls describe treating 81 different diseases using myrrh and honey. Myrrh essential oil is still known for its ability to clear up infections of the skin and throat.

When King Tut's tomb was opened in 1922, there were more than 50 alabaster jars used for essential oils. The oils were gone, and only traces were left behind. Some stores of gold were undisturbed, and it is assumed that the grave robbers valued the essential oils above gold.

Ancient Chinese medical practitioners passed down their knowledge of essential oils used for curing common illnesses and calming down disturbed minds. They dip their acupuncture needles in essential oils for a deeper sense of healing.

Indian medics have used herbs and aromatic plants in their Ayurvedic medicinal system for thousands of years. They distilled essential oils to use in massage therapy and left recipes for essential oils that provide medical enhancements.

The Greeks followed the ways of the Egyptians and the most well-known physician of that time, Hippocrates, was a firm believer in holistic medicine and aromatherapy massage. It is believed that Hippocrates stopped a plague in Athens by using essential oils. In ancient Greece, Dioscorides wrote a book that described methods still used by aromatherapists today. Essential oils were extensively used to purify public buildings in opening ceremonies, and were essential elements in steam baths.

The Arabian empire drew on the Greek and Roman experiences and uses of essential oils. The Persian physician Avicenna was credited with perfecting the distillation process of essential oils in 1037 Ad.

Arabian traders used frankincense essential oil as a commodity. Frankincense was and is very expensive and was often valued more than gold.

During the Black Plague of the 17th century, essential oils, specifically lavender, was spread over the floors of the castles and individuals fastened bunches of lavender to their wrists to protect themselves. Lavender is a known insect repellent and wards off mosquitos. Those who wore lavender may have escaped the Black Plague since mosquitos were culprits in spreading Black Plague. Lavender stops mosquitos from biting.

By the late 1800s, the active elements of natural remedies were isolated, and essential oils began their modern comeback. Dr. Rene-Maurice Gattefosse, Ph.D., a French chemist, began studying essential oils in 1907. In 1910, Dr. Gattefosse was terribly burned in a laboratory accident. He plunged his hands into a vat of lavender, and the lavender solution stopped the gasification of the tissue. He began studying essential oils and their properties in earnest and is now credited with being the father of aromatherapy.

Essential oils were used during World War I by Dr. Monciere. He used essential oils for their wound-healing and antibacterial properties. He also developed different types of aromatic ointments to ease the pain and suffering among the soldiers.

Dr. Jean Valnet, a colleague of Dr. Gattefosse, practiced medicine in Tonkin, China during WWII. Dr. Valnet exhausted his supply of antibiotics and began using therapeutic-grade essential oils on soldiers' injuries. To his glee and surprise, these essential oils actually combated and counteracted infection. He saved the lives of numerous soldiers who might have otherwise died of wound infection and inflammation. The work of Dr. Valnet was carried on by two of his students who further broke down and wrote about the anti-viral, antibacterial, antifungal and antiseptic properties of essential oils.

The 1980s led to the rediscovery of essential oils in the United States. The role that essential oils play in combating present-day diseases is being researched and believers are using essential oils more than ever.

Today there are numerous massage clinics that blend their own essential oils and deeply believe in the healing power of massage and essential oil application.

Elements

Essential oils are those wonderful, but volatile or somewhat unpredictable liquids made naturally in plants. All parts of the plant may be used to extract essential oils including the leaves, stems, roots, flowers, fruit, seeds, and bark. Technically, essential oils are not oils at all but highly concentrated plant components. The determining factors of the transparency and beneficial values of an essential oil is in its chemical and organic compounds. These compounds come about due to a number of factors. These features include the stems, flowers, bark or root of the plant where the oil is produced, soil conditions, organic or chemical fertilizers, climate, altitude harvest season, geographic regions and distillation processes.

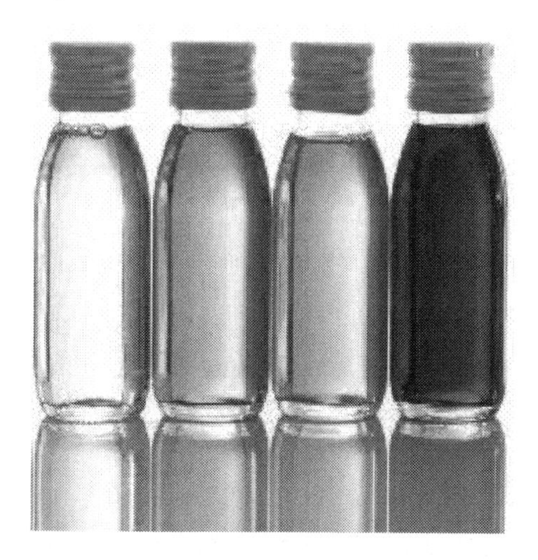

Essential oils - bottles

Essential oils include plants' immune-strengthening, regenerating, and oxygenating properties. The oils are lipid-soluble and can penetrate cell walls to bring immunity, oxygenating, and regenerating properties into the heart of the cell. Essential oils can penetrate cells in the body within twenty minutes. Oil penetration provides oxygenation and healing to all cells in the body.

The molecules of essential oils are miniscule, easily absorbed through the skin, and contain the perfect ingredients for use in personal care items. Essential oils heal the body, soften the skin, and nourish the cells. Essential oils will not build up and become toxic in your body. Essential oils will heal where they need to heal and move on through your body.

One of the most powerful ingredients in essential oils are antioxidants that provide an unfriendly environment for free radicals. Free radicals are those raving molecules that are responsible for aging, diseases and tissue damage. Certain essential oils prevent free radical damage as well as mutations, fungus, and oxidation within the cells. It is a bit unnerving to think that cells can build up fungus and mutations, but these are the harbingers of diseases. Science proves that essential oils cleanse the cells and blood in the body, and act as antibacterial, anticancer, antifungal, and antiseptic fighters.

The heterogenetic benefits of essential oils depend on the chemical constitution and the amount of chemicals in proportion to other properties. Science has proven there are many individual oils containing 200 to 800 different chemical components. What an essential oil does depends on the chemical reactions in the host plant.

A main centerpiece of essential oils are the sesquiterpenes, or the substances that pass the blood-brain barrier and slow the progression of diseases such as Alzheimer's, Lou Gehrig's, and Parkinson's. This component also eases the symptoms and heartache of multiple sclerosis. Sesquiterpenes in essential oils erase or rewrite the miswritten codes in DNA. In addition, essential oils are highly effective in easing the symptoms of cancer and perhaps actually stopping the growth of debilitating cancer tumors.

Scientists have discovered that certain essential oils can move through the blood-brain barrier, and the high levels of sesquiterpenes in these oils increase the amount of oxygen in the limbic system of the brain. The result is an increase in secretions of antibodies, neurotransmitters, and endorphins.

In 1989, the amygdala, a gland in the limbic system, was discovered to be a major player in emotions. Stimulating this gland with fragrance is a key that can unlock and release emotional trauma. Perhaps this is why a bath infused with essential oils is so therapeutic, stress relieving and relaxing.

Essential oils also include oxygenated compounds labeled as ketones, alcohols, phenols, oxides, and esters. Oxygenated compounds are anti-fungal, calming and relaxing. They fight infections and have a sedative effect on the central nervous system.

The phenol compounds in essential oils are responsible for the fragrance. They are antiseptic, but their stimulating compounds but are a bit caustic to the skin. Some of the more caustic essential oils are clove and cinnamon. Do not apply these oils directly to the skin. Be careful when using oregano and thyme essential oils, as they can cause rashes when applied 'neat' to the skin.

Aromatherapists apply essential oils in carriers directly to the skin using aromatherapy massage, but oils are also used to freshen the air via diffusers or sprays. You can inhale the oils directly, but be careful not to swallow or consume certain liquid oils.

Watch for other essential oils that should never be used undiluted on skin. Read the cautionary labels and combine these oils with carrier oils, butters, alcohols, or waxes.

Lavender and chamomile essential oils can be applied directly to wounds and the skin without dilution. It only takes a few drops of these oils to provide the needed relief.

Extracting Methods

Distillation

There are many ways to separate the essential oils from the plant matter. Ways include effleurage, expressed oils, (cold-pressed), team distillation, solvent extraction, fractional distillation, D-percolations, carbon dioxide extraction and the phytonic process.

Enfleurage is the oldest method of extracting essential oils, but is not used due to high costs. It involves lying flower petals on a glass sheet that is spread with a thin layer of fat. The flowers are pressed between another sheet of glass and the essential oils diffuse into the fat. The fat is collected and the oils are extracted using alcohol. This is a very time-consuming process and highly labor-intensive.

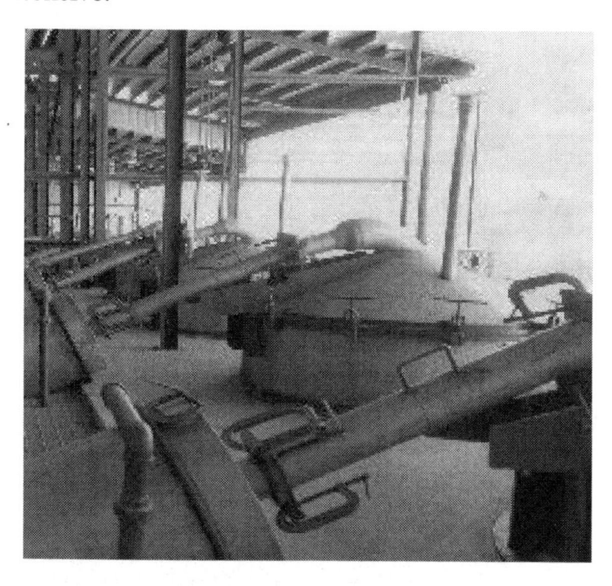

Essential Oil Distillation

Water distillation involves, of course, water. The botanic material is immersed in water, and the still is brought to a boil.

This method protects the oils, and the water acts as a barrier to prevent the botanic materials from overheating.

After the condensed material cools down, the water and essential oils are separated, and the oils are emptied into sterile vessels.

This water that is leached off is referred to as plant water essence. The water is often sold as a component for use in other fragrant products. Popular plant water essences include rose, lavender, lemon balm, clary sage and orange blossom.

Water, steam, hydrodiffusion, and water and steam distillation all involve heat. Great care needs to be taken with extraction. The temperature and length of exposure to heat must be just right to prevent damage to the oils.

Steam distillation has been used for hundreds of years and is one of the best ways to extract essential oils. This is a method releasing the aromatic molecules from the plant material. The steam opens the pockets where the oils reside in the plant materials. The molecules of volatile oils escape from the plant and evaporate into the steam.

The temperature of the steam must be carefully controlled. Just enough steam needs to force the plant to let go of the oils, yet cannot be too hot, so as not to burn the plant material.

The next step is to condense the steam, form a liquid, and separate the water and essential oil. Steam is produced at a pressure greater than the atmosphere and boils at 100°C. Boiling facilitates the removal of the essential oils from the plant material at a fast rate to prevent damage to the oil. For example, lavender is heat-sensitive and with steam distillation the vital essential oil is not damaged.

Essential oil distilling steam equipment includes the condenser, separator and cooking chambers. This equipment comes together to impact the equality of the oil. Steam distillation is the best way to produce therapeutic-grade oils.

Hydrodiffusion is also steam distillation. The difference between regular steam and hydro steam diffusion is how the steam is introduced. Hydro comes from the top, and traditional steam methods are from the bottom. Hydro steam distillation uses less steam, has a shorter processing time and yields more essential oils.

Expression is a method of extracting essential oils that are cold-pressed. There is no heat used in this process. Nut and seed oils plus citrus peels are extracted using a cold pressed method. The oils are forced from the plant material under high pressure.

The quality of essential oil that is produced by cold-pressing or expression is high. Some manufacturers feel that the oil needs to be further refined by adding chemicals or high heat.

Solvent

Solvent processing is done by soaking the flowers in hot oil to rupture cell membranes. The hot oil or solvent absorbs the essence. The oils or solvent is cleared from the botanicals and decanted. This is the way the perfume industry receives their oils. Oils extracted via solvents are not therapeutic-grade.

There are flowers that have too little volatile oil to express and chemical components cannot be extracted via distillation methods. A solvent like hexane or supercritical carbon dioxide is used to move the oils from the plants. Using supercritical carbon dioxide extracts the waxes and essential oils. Further processing with liquid carbon dioxide separates the waxes from the essential oils. This low temperature prevents the decomposition and denaturing of compounds. When the oils and waxes are extracted, the pressure is reduced, and carbon dioxide reverts to a gas. This modern method does produce a high-quality oil, but it is very cost-prohibitive.

Florasol extraction is ozone-friendly, but it does pose significant danger to the environment if large quantities are used. This process is banned in Europe, but one advantage of Florasol extraction is the pure essential oils that result from it.

Any way you extract the essential oils is expensive. It takes up to 5,000 pounds of rose petals to yield one pound of rose essential oil. Almost 1,000 pounds of jasmine or about 3 million flowers are needed to yield a pound of jasmine essential oil. Lavender requires at least 200 pounds of flowers to make a pound of lavender essential oil.

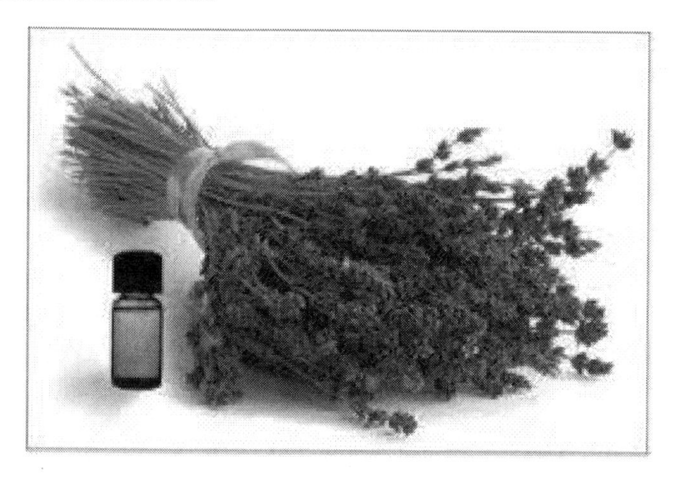

Reflexology - palmbeachgardens-chiropractor.com

Chapter 2

How to Use Essential Oils

"Practitioners of aromatherapy believe that fragrances in the oils stimulate nerves in the nose. Those nerves send impulses to the part of the brain that controls memory and emotion. Depending on the type of oil or the scent, the results on the body may be calming or stimulating."

—WebMD.com

Your sense of smell impacts your feelings of well-being, emotion, and mood. The human brain can distinguish about 10,000 different scents and most of these scents directly affect how we act and feel. Essential oils are all about the smell, touch, and feel. They offer health benefits and feelings of well-being that include:

- Stress relief
- Relaxation
- Mood enhancing

- Balance and well-being
- Relief of minor discomfort
- Immune, respiratory and circulatory system boosts.

If you are looking for a natural way to feel good and stay healthy, before you purchase essential oils, there are nine safety items you should look for:

Watch for the term "pure." You are looking for therapeutic-grade oils rather than "pure."

- There are preparations that are synthetic fragrances. Certain oils do not exist in a natural state, and these are a combination of essential oils, synthetics, and absolutes. Honeysuckle, linden, gardenia and frangipani are examples of synthetic fragrances. These fragrances are wonderful but will not give you the healthy properties of genuine essential oils.
- Watch for oils that are impure. Research has discovered that the more expensive an "essential" oil is, the greater the risk of adulteration or contamination.
- There are many levels of buyers and suppliers in the essential oil industry. The more levels you must go through to purchase an essential oil creates a greater risk of contamination. Buy oils directly from the distiller to ensure you are purchasing pure, therapeutic essential oils.

- Watch out for expressed citrus oils that may contain pesticide residues. Citrus is a natural pesticide, and often distillers add chemicals to heighten their bug-repelling qualities.

- Look out for low grades of essential oils sold as "pure." One essential oil that marketers seem to sell in low-grade volumes is ylang-ylang.

- Avoid extenders in essential oils. Expensive oils are often drawn-out with jojoba oil, or other solvents to make the oils flow easier or pour from a jar. Purchase essential oils that drop, not pour.

- Bulking is a problem. Bulking is post-distillation combining of oils from one essential oil to another. Bulking is practiced to make the products cheaper or make the essential oil conform to some standard in the fragrance industry. Purchase blends from a reputable dealer or make your own unique blends.

- Aromatherapy or the use of essential oils is a complementary health treatment. It is not a replacement for traditional medical practices or prescription medication, but it is effective at alleviating the discomfort associated with ill health. Oils are very helpful for some cases, supportive in others, and may have little or no effect in other situations. Oils are not meant to treat or cure serious medical conditions, but to calm down and provide added benefits to conventional medical procedures.

Choosing the right essential oil depends on the purpose. If you want to elevate your mood or you are treating a wound, there are different essential oils for those tasks. There is not exact list that specifies which essential oils treat which health concern. You can use several different types of essential oils to manage the same problem. Be proactive and research, talk to quality aromatherapists, and perhaps experiment just a little, following suggestions and rules, of course.

Apply essential oils to the skin, inhale the fragrance or ingest the oils. The application method depends on the desired effect and the oil you select. Note that there are some essential oils that are irritating to the skin because of chemistry and other oils that are rubbed into your skin to provide health and calming benefits. A good rule of thumb is:

- Wound care involves topical applications.
- Use topical or inhalation methods to change moods. If you need to affect your mood quickly, inhale directly from the bottle.
- Baths can involve inhalation and topical absorption.

Safety

Safety is a major concern of reputable distillers of essential oils. When used properly essential oils are beneficial and very safe.

Amateurs do like to experiment and can hurt themselves by using highly concentrated botanical substances improperly. Beware of using essential oils internally, dilute with a carrier oil before using on your skin, keep out of the reach of children, and avoid contact with eyes and mucous membranes. Do not use citrus oils on your skin when outside exposing your body to UV light. Use only pure essential oils. By all means, side-step synthetic fragrances. Do not use essential oils on infants, children, pregnant women, the elderly or those with serious health problems unless you know what you are doing. Store essential and carrier oils in dark glass bottles to prevent spoilage.

Topical use of essential oils involves diluting an oil in a carrier substance. You can use vegetable or nut oil or even water. Use a concentration no more than 3-5%. Three drops of pure essential oil dropped into one teaspoon (5cc) of carrier is the general dilution amount. Make sure you shake the bottle to mix the carrier and oil together. Massage using essential oils usually calls for a 1% solution or 1 drop of essential oils into a carrier. When using massage therapy for infants, use a 0.25% solution and 0.5% for toddlers.

Purchase pure carrier oils in natural health food stores. Preferred carriers are cold-pressed and organic oils. Examples of carrier oils include sweet almond oil, apricot kernel oil, jojoba oil, grape seed oil or avocado. These oils do not have strong smells of their own and mix nicely with any essential oil. Do keep your oils in the refrigerator and tightly lidded. They will keep for up to a year; however, if they smell rancid, throw them out immediately.

Wound care requires that the oil be very gentle to the skin and have an antimicrobial property. Lavender essential oil is one of the few oils that can be used undiluted on small areas of the skin. Touch gently to minor cuts using a clean cloth. Lavender helps wounds and burns heal quickly. Chamomile is also an excellent "neat" topical essential oil. You can apply lavender or chamomile directly to the skin with a cotton ball or cloth.

Topical Applications

Compresses

Dilute essential oils in a liquid carrier and apply to a dressing. Clean and soft clothes work the best. Apply the dressing directly to the affected area. The compress can be warm or cool; whatever feels best. Add a few drops of ginger essential oil to the water being used as the carrier. Soak a soft, clean cloth in the solution and place on a stiff joint, or a head, neck, arm, leg, hand, belly, back or anyplace you are feeling achy and need relief.

Compresses are very safe methods of using essential oils. Apply compresses as long and as often as you like for almost any type of concern.

Cold compresses are effective in relieving the itching and pain of insect bites. Use 3-4 drops of lavender and 1-3 drops of eucalyptus in the cold water, wet a cloth, wring and apply directly to the bug bite.

Cold compresses help relieve headaches. Lavender is the perfect essential oil for headaches, but you can also use peppermint and eucalyptus. Just a few drops of any of these oils in a bowl of water, soak your cloth and lay the cloth over your face. Breathing in the essential oil fragrance and using the cool cloth is a soothing way to get rid of simple headaches.

Hot compresses are used for pus-producing wounds. Add a drop or two of thyme and or oregano essential oils to hot water. Dip your cloth in the water, wring out, and place over the infected area. You can safely apply this compress every three to four hours.

Warm compresses are perfect for chest congestion. The best essential oil to use for congestion is eucalyptus. This essential oil has a distinctive taste and odor and is a stimulating decongestant. Apply the warm eucalyptus compress to your chest and breathe deeply. You will have the benefits of the aroma of eucalyptus plus the warmth of the compress.

Cool compresses are great for reducing fevers. Use a few drops of lavender, eucalyptus, peppermint or chamomile in cool water. Place a cloth on the forehead. The smells are heavenly, and the cool relief is very welcomed.

If you experience hot flashes from being hot on very warm days or are experiencing hormonal changes, use a few drops of peppermint or spearmint on a cool cloth. Drape over the back of your neck. Rub down your arms and legs with the mixture and even apply to your face.

Massage

Using essential oils with a carrier oil for a deep massage is a wonderful way to maximize the healing power of the oils. Massage can have a calming or energizing effect, and it all depends on the oils you chose. It is important to dilute essential oils with a carrier oil prior to the massage. When combining essential oils used in massage, employ good quality carrier oils, and store the mixture in a dark bottle. You can mix any combination of oils you like, but do be aware that they can turn rancid fairly quickly. Store in a cool, dark container with the lid tightly closed.

Massage helps improve flexibility, mobility, and circulation. It reduces stress and eases tension, and can take away the pain of headaches and migraines, cramps, and spasms. Using essential oils in massage improves the immune system by stimulating the limbic system and releasing toxins.

Using essential oils in combination with massage is the ultimate in luxury and healing. Combine well-chosen essential oils with a carrier to promote relaxation, reduce stress, and improve circulation. Massage plus essential oils can also reduce swelling and pain.

There are essential oils that act as aphrodisiacs or substances that enhance or stimulate passion and arousal. Create an intimate mood by using massage and the accompanying essential oils.

For a massage to alleviate stress, blend six drops of clary sage, two drops of lemon and three drops of lavender. For sleep-inducing or anti-inflammatory massages, use five drops of Roman chamomile, and five drops of lavender. If you have sore muscles, massage in two drops of ginger, one drop of black pepper, four drops of peppermint, and five drops of eucalyptus.

The perfect aphrodisiac blend of massage oil is eight drops of sandalwood and two drops of jasmine, all mixed in a very nice carrier oil.

Mix the oils well and store in the usual airtight and dark glass container. You only need to use a small amount, up to one teaspoon, for each massage.

Foot Massage

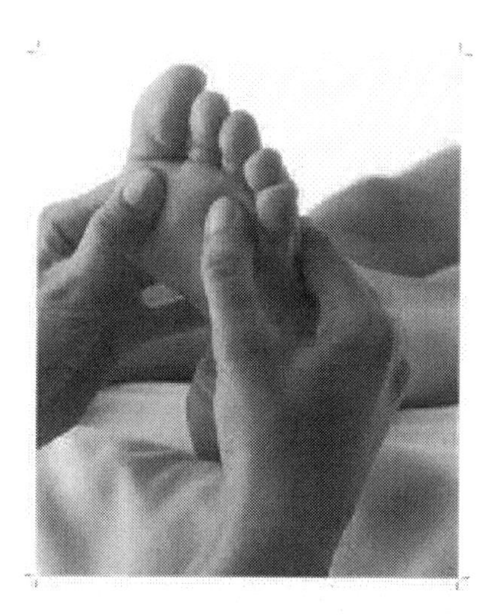

Become a believer in regular foot massage. The feet are the passageways to the body. Massaging the feet can bring improvements to health and relieve stress and anxiety. There are many disorders that have roots in emotions and working on your feet can reach those deep hidden blockages and move them out of your life. Professionals who are certified in acupuncture, reflexology and foot zoning use specific trigger points on the feet to check for problems and weaknesses in different systems of the body.

All day, your feet bear the weight of your body. Feet are encased in shoes and never touched or given any attention. No wonder there are more blockages on your feet than in any other reflex area. Believe it or not, you will get better healing results from a good foot massage than any other type of massage.

Combining foot massage with essential oils provides double the health-giving pleasure. Try blending myrrh and frankincense in a carrier oil. These two oils are used to enhance the immune system. Myrrh is a calming essential oil and frankincense is an oil used for anxiety, stress, depression, fears, and nightmares.

Soaking in a Tub

Easing into a bath is one of the most wonderful ways to relax. Ancient Romans knew that jumping into a tub for a soak was the cure for any horrible day. Healers in Japan have known for thousands of years that just 10 minutes of soaking in a bath improves your attitude and responses to physical and mental stressors.

Add geranium to your bath water to neutralize out-of-control emotions. Pink grapefruit essential oil provides mental clarity, and rose essential oils have skin-enhancing properties. Add three to four drops of these essential oils to bath water and gently mix the water. Soaking gives you a wonderful absorption through the skin. Try adding one teaspoon of bergamot to lower your blood pressure while stimulating your feel-good hormones. Add clary sage to bring you peace of mind when you are feeling agitated. Inhale the volatilized essential oils as you bathe. Use a few tablespoons of full cream as a dispersant. You now have the added benefit of essential oils and a milk bath.

Overdosed on caffeine during the day? Take a bath with Bulgarian rose otto oil. This oil has a zesty smell that gives your senses a blast, and draws impurities out of your skin. You can also try jojoba oils packed with energizing B vitamins. Mix the two together, and you have created a wonderful wake-up call.

Do something nice for yourself. Add a few drops of eucalyptus oil to your bath. Eucalyptus essential oil combats exhaustion and anxiety. It relaxes your overworked blood vessels. Breathe the fragrance of eucalyptus in and close your eyes for a minute or two.

Note that essential oils are not water soluble. They will float on top of the water, and your skin is exposed to the full strengths of the essential oils. Use a carrier. Bath salts work well, or mix two portions of Epsom salts and one part baking soda to three measures of sea salt. Stir in six drops of an essential oil and mix into your bath water. Lavender works very nice in this mix or choose any essential oil you enjoy.

Ingesting

Internal applications of essential oils require supervision. Ask your healthcare provider or an aromatherapist which oils can be ingested without injury.

Gargling or drinking some types of essential oils can help you calm down or cure a sore throat. Mix one drop of tea tree oil in a glass of water and gargle for sore throat discomfort. Do not swallow the mixture, just spit it out.

Drop in a couple of drops of lemon essential oil to your water bottle, shake, add ice, and drink. You do not need expensive water additives that add chemicals to your body.

The FDA (Federal Drug Administration) has approved some essential oils for internal use. These oils are designated as GRAS or recognized as safe for human consumption. Oils without this designation should never be ingested.

Capsules are the most convenient and common ways to take essential oils internally. Just place 1-10 drops of essential oil inside a capsule, seal it and swallow. You can fill the capsule with olive oil if you feel uneasy ingesting undiluted essential oils.

It is also very easy to use essential oils internally by adding them to beverages. Place a drop of essential oil in 1-4 cups of rice milk, almond milk or water. Then drink and enjoy.

Essential oils can are used in cooking. Just remember you only need a few drops of the very concentrated essential oil. Try adding three drops of wild orange essential oil to cream cheese icing. You will be amazed at the taste and texture. You can also add lemon or peppermint to icings, cakes, or breads. Use essential oils in salad dressings. You only need a few drops to make an exquisite dressing.

Some essential oils can be used internally for vaginal insertion. Oils can be diluted in 2-3 teaspoons of a carrier oils and used with a vaginal syringe. Hold the oils in place with a tampon. You can also soak the tampon in the oil and carrier mixture and insert it as you normally would. Using essential oils, this way helps with vaginal dryness, yeast infections, and general soreness.

Rectal insertion is often recommended to aid in healing various internal conditions. Use a rectal syringe to place in capsules in your rectum or use as a suppository.

The antibacterial properties of essential oils are very effective when used in the dishwasher, clothes washer or clothes dryer. Add two drops of lemon essential oil to dishwater for an awesome-smelling kitchen and sparkling dishes. Use lemon oil or white fir oil on a cloth when you are dusting.

Inhaling

Inhaling essential oils through your nose and into your respiratory tract allows the concentration of essential oils to flow through the blood stream. The fragrance activates the centers of the brain that govern your moods, emotions and enhance immune functions. The easiest and most direct way to use essential oils at any time is to take the cap off the bottle and inhale. You can also use 3-4 drops of lavender or chamomile on a handkerchief and breathe deeply. Breathing essential oils through a handkerchief was a favorite way to inhale essential oils during the 1900s.

Use commercial aromatherapy inhalers. Just carry your inhaler in your purse and use when needed. Inhale essential oils by adding 5-6 drops to a steaming bowl of water, place a cover over your head and inhale the steam.

Oil diffusers are safe and very effective in dispersing essential oils into the environment. Use ¼ teaspoon of oil diluted with water and add to the dispenser. Inhale the tiny oil molecules as they float in the air. Add rosemary to your diffuser for mental stimulation, and drop in lavender essential oil for relaxation.

Diffusers pass a continuous stream of air over the oil source. This stream creates an evaporated mist without heating the oil. If you do not have an essential oil diffuser, you can also add a few drops of essential oils to water in a small bowl and burn it over a candle.

Never directly burn essential oils. Do not use essential oils in an incense burner. Essential oils have a chemical structure that changes, and not for the better, when burned.

Go slow when diffusing essential oils. Start with a few drops and gradually build up to a higher strength. If you notice a mild headache coming on or you have a nauseated feeling, you may need to turn off your diffuser.

Cold and hay fever sufferers are comforted by using eucalyptus or peppermint oil in your diffuser. You will immediately see a huge difference in your breathing. A diffuser will also work as a pickme-up at the end of a long work day. Add lemon, sage, peppermint, grapefruit and make a blend soothe your stressed brain.

Take a trip to the sauna and enhance your experience by mixing ten drops of eucalyptus or juniper essential oil in a pint of water. Place the mixture onto the heat source of the sauna. You will get an awesome cleansing and detoxifying effect on your body.

Spraying

Try adding drops of different types of essential oil to a fine-misting spray bottle. If you are feeling earthy, use patchouli, frankincense and cedar. Essential oils are highly personal and mood enhancing, and what you love today may be something you dislike tomorrow.

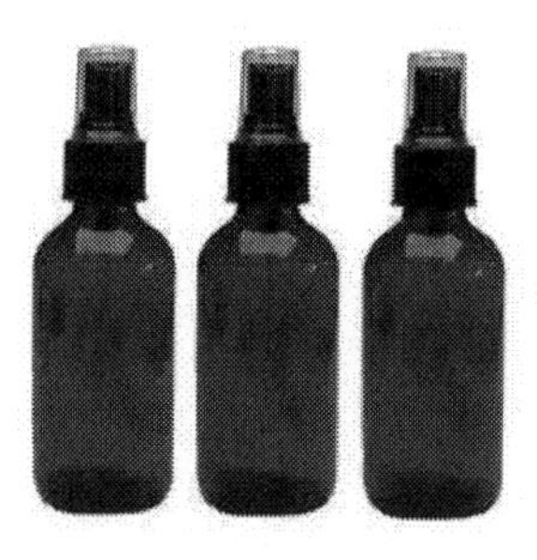

Essential oil spray bottle

Spraying essential oils is a very good way to deodorize a room or set a mood. Add oils to a water or alcohol based solution, pour into a spray bottle, shake and spray away. You might want to try an aqueous solution of pine or citrus for a Christmas-like mood. Try peppermint oil to stimulate alertness.

Keep a bottle of sprayable essential oils in every room of your home: one by your bed as a linen spray, one on your desk to keep you alert, and one in the living room as a general air freshener.

Take a small spray bottle with a fine mister and add an ounce of good vodka, purified water or mix alcohol and water together. Add 20 drops of your favorite essential oil or blend. Combine the ingredients in a spray bottle, shake well and spray needed to achieve the desired effect or mood.

For night time calming, use 15 drops of chamomile and five drops of lavender or you can use ten drops of chamomile, five drops of sage, and five drops of bergamot. Ten drops of rosemary and ten drops of lavender is also very nice to use when you are trying to go to sleep.

Need energy? Use 12 drops of rosemary and eight drops bergamot in a spray bottle. Ten drops of peppermint and ten drops of lemon essential oil, or ten drops of bergamot, five drops of orange and five drops of grapefruit will put a spring in you step. Spray it around the room. You might try spraying it in the office to give all your colleagues a lift.

For those with depressed or blue feelings, 12 drops of orange essential oil plus eight drops of grapefruit oil, or even just 20 drops of grapefruit sprayed around the room will lighten up your mood.

Steaming

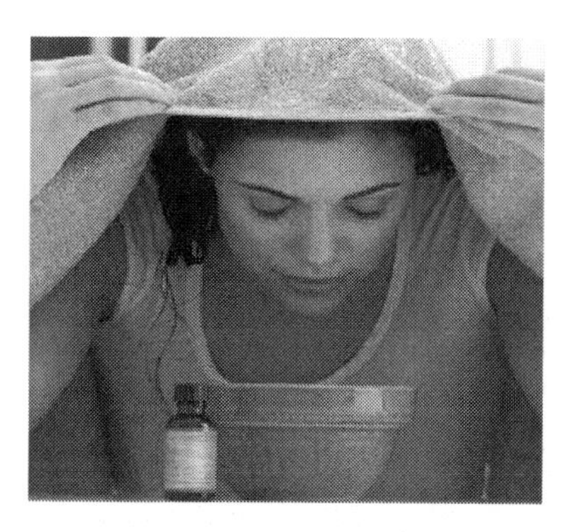

Remedies for Allergies and Congestion.

Steaming essential oils will help with respiratory issues. Do not use this method, however, if you are asthmatic. Eucalyptus, cedarwood, and pine are particularly helpful if you have a sinus infection. Place several drops of an essential oil in a bowl of steaming water. Place a towel over your head, bend over the bowl and breathe deeply. This is a very potent method of using essential oils to clear your sinuses. Start with only 1-2 drops, or you might be overwhelmed. Add more drops of essential oils if you can tolerate it. Do keep your eyes shut to avoid getting the essential oil fumes into your eyes.

Use steaming for bronchitis and add basil, benzoin, clove and frankincense to your bowl. Make your personal mixture that gives you the most relief. Keep a copy of the proportions you need in your medicine cabinet.

Pesky colds do well with a steam of bay, black pepper, clove, ginger, or myrrh. Use rosemary, tea tree and orange essential oils, and cyprus to control coughing.

Dry Evaporation

Dry evaporation is a good way to disperse essential oils. You simply place drops of essential oil on a cotton ball or tissue and let the scent evaporate into the air. If you need an intense dose, sniff the cotton ball. You can keep the cotton ball or tissue on your desk to keep the air around you smelling awesome and to improve your mood or work habits.

Chapter 3

Therapeutic Uses of Essential Oils

"Bad smells. Bad memories. That's because the memory is right next to the smell box inside your brain. Nothing makes you remember like a smell."

—*The Mentalist*

Essential oils smell wonderful, but they are even better when used as a therapeutic tool. Think about your favorite smells. A memory probably pops up, and some scents can actually improve your health. "Essential oils can have a healing effect mentally, physically, and emotionally," said Brianna Scarpello, a marketer and expert on essential oils.

Essential oils are antiseptic. Being antiseptic is one of their most valuable properties. Antiseptics include anti-viral, anti-fungal, anti-bacterial and general anti-microbial activity. Lemon, tea tree, garlic, eucalyptus, thyme, pine, lavender, eucalyptus, and sandalwood are examples of some popular essential oils with high antiseptic properties.

Lemon and orange essential oils come from the peels of the fruit and have powerful anti-microbial properties. These properties are used to destroy pathogenic bacteria, viruses, and fungi. Lemon and orange essential oils contain concentrated forms of citrus bioflavonoids known as vitamin P. Vitamin P improves microcirculation, enhances tissue oxygenation, and functions as an antioxidant.

Many essential oils have anti-inflammatory properties that help take away the symptoms of swelling and tenderness, pain, redness, and partial or total loss of tissue function. Oils that are considered highly anti-inflammatory are chamomile, lavender, rose, benzoin, myrrh, and sandalwood. Benzoin is one of the lesser-known essential oils and comes from the Benzoin tree. Use benzoin as an antidepressant plus an anti-inflammatory agent.

Restoring tissue function and rejuvenation of cells are functions of pine, rosemary, and basil. These essential oils are also used to restore the adrenal glands. Jasmine, cypress, and ylang-ylang reestablish functions of the reproductive glands, and lavender and chamomile regenerate cells in the skin.

Essential oils have a pronounced effect on the nervous system. They produce relaxation, pain relief, and help relieve muscle spasms. Oils that are beneficial as sedatives are lavender, neroli, rose, geranium, benzoin, and ylang-ylang.

When searching for essential oils to use in healing, look for high quality therapeutic-grade oils that are pure, medicinal and steam distilled. Avoid essential warehouse oils; go for the best quality you can.

Some Oils for Healing

Essential oils contain important medicinal properties. They should be a part of a natural medicine cabinet. Essential oils work to support the body's healing system and when used correctly are wonderful complements to medical healing.

A very nice all-around essential oil is lavender. It is a gorgeous plant and just smelling lavender promotes a feeling of calm and peace. Lavender oil comes from the actual flower and not the leaves or seeds. Lavender essential oils are antiseptic and awesome for cleaning cuts, healing sores, burns and other wounds. Lavender is known to help reduce pain. It is perfect for decreasing anxiety and other nervous conditions. Spray lavender around a room when you are taking care of an anxious patient, and they quickly calm down.

Clove and cinnamon essential oils are also high in antioxidant properties. Two drops of clove and four drops of cinnamon have the antioxidant capacity of five pounds of carrots, 2.5 quarts of carrot juice, 20 ounces of orange juice or 10 oranges.

Clove essential oil holds the health benefits of antimicrobial, antifungal and antiseptic. It is also a great aphrodisiac. Use it for coughs, asthma, tooth issues, and blood impurities.

Cinnamon enhances insulin receptor site activity. It reduces the amount of insulin in the bloodstream and contributes to a stable blood sugar, helps with fat metabolism and decreases cellular inflammation. Cinnamon essential oils are also powerful, antimicrobial, and have immune-boosting properties.

Essential Oils and Common Ailments

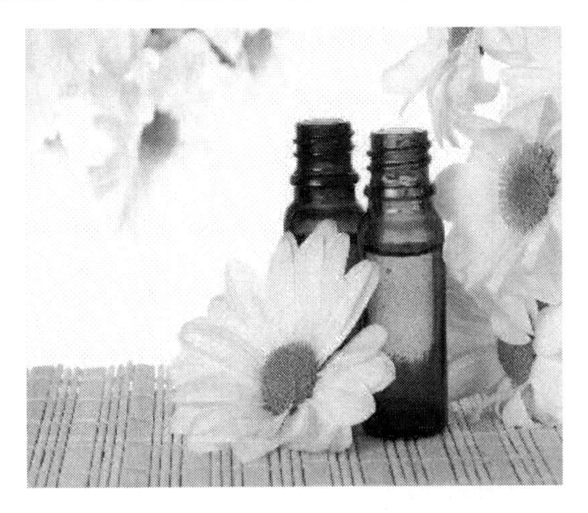

Essential Oils

Essential oils can be used to help with psychological conditions of ADD/ADHD. Characterized by inattentiveness, restlessness, and concentration issues, ADD/ADHD can be helped by combining equal parts of basil and lavender. Use them through a diffuser or apply a mixture of three drops to the crown of the head. You can use this blend by applying 1-3 drops on the bottoms of the feet and massaging stress points.

Massage and aromatherapy provide valuable support to people suffering from AIDS and related illnesses. Those with AIDS suffer from the mental anguish of being diagnosed with HIV. Inhaling essential oil vapors using room diffusers, oil burners or warm water can help ease the stress. Add oils to baths, footbaths, Sitz baths, and douches. Use direct application of essential oils when diluted for skin ailments. Use in massage for all-over body relaxation.

Many teens suffer from acne or a skin condition characterized by red and irritated blemishes on the skin. Acne is found on the oil-producing parts of the body like the face, back, chest and back of the neck. Clear up skin by using geranium, sandalwood, thyme, lemon, lemongrass, marjoram, and patchouli essential oils. Dilute as recommended in a carrier. You can use any of these essential oils in a spray mist to help keep your skin refreshed during the day.

Those who suffer from high blood pressure or hypertension will benefit from using lemon, ylang-ylang, marjoram, eucalyptus, lavender, clove, clary sage, lemon, and wintergreen. You can add several drops of any of these oils in a bath to give you a stress relieving session and to lower your blood pressure. Mix five drops of geranium, eight drops of lemongrass oil, and three drops of lavender in a carrier oil like fractionated coconut oil. Gently rub over your heart and reflex points on the left foot and hand. Feel the stress melt away.

Winter is bronchitis season and symptoms of this inflammation include coughing, breathlessness, thick phlegm, and fatigue. Give relief to the bronchitis sufferer by diffusing into the air a mixture of eucalyptus, thyme, white fir, basil, clary sage, cypress, tea tree oil, peppermint, rosemary, wintergreen, and myrrh. You can also apply the oils to your hands, tissues or cotton balls and inhale. Try diluting the oils as recommend and applying to your chest, sinuses, neck, and reflex points on the feet.

If you are suffering from canker sores, the small round sores that develop in the mouth, you can ease the pain by using tea tree oil, oregano, Roman chamomile, and myrrh. Just dilute with carrier oil or water and apply one drop to the canker location.

Diaper rash is a nuisance to mother and babies. You can solve the rash problems by using essential oils. Blend one drop of Roman chamomile and one drop of lavender oils with one teaspoon fractionated coconut oil. Apply to the sore rash area. It will feel great almost instantly.

Irritable bowel syndrome is an intestinal disorder characterized by diarrhea, gas, constipation, and bloating, cramping, and abdominal pain. It is a very common disorder and also very painful. You can feel much better if you add two drops of peppermint oil and two drops of Chamomile to eight ounces of distilled water and drink at least 1-2 times a day. You can also place two drops of these oils in an empty capsule and swallow. It will feel great to your sore and tired tummy if you dilute 1-2 drops in fractionated coconut oil and apply over the abdomen and then use a hot compress.

If you have difficulty falling or staying asleep, essential oils can be the answer for you. Stress, medications, drug or alcohol use, anxiety and depression are just some of the causes of insomnia. Combine 6 drops of orange with six drops of lavender. Apply this blend to big toes, and bottoms of your feet. Put a couple of drops around the navel and three drops on the back of the neck. You can also combine two drops of Roman chamomile, six drops of geranium, three drops of lemon, and four drops of sandalwood and a good carrier oil in a dark glass bottle. Shake to mix and add six drops of this mixture to your bath before bedtime. Add a little more power to your sleep and spray lavender essential oil on your pillow. Spraying lavender should do the trick and cure your insomnia.

When teeth hurt, your entire body hurts. You may have an infected tooth or an abscess or a cavity that is growing more damaging. Leaving your infected tooth alone will cause swelling of the face, swollen lymph nodes, and a fever. If an abscess ruptures, it will leave a foul-tasting liquid in your mouth, and if left untreated it will spread to other areas of your neck and jaw. Before you can get to the dentist, you might want to use clove oil, helichrysum, tea tree oil, frankincense, chamomile or wintergreen on the abscess. Use any of these or a mixture of several as a compress and apply to the affected area. You can use clove or peppermint oil by applying one or two drops to a cotton ball and applying to the gums in the area of the toothache.

Ear Care and Essential Oils

Takin care of ears with essential oils will provide your family with a safe and sure way to keep ear infections at a minimum. Mix five drops of lavender, five drops of geranium and five drops of melaleuca in one tablespoon of coconut oil. Clean your ear with a natural cleaner and use a Q-tip to rub the essential oils mixture around the inside of your ear. Do not put the Q-tip in your ear so far that you cannot see the tip. Do this twice a day if you have an ear infection.

If you are going camping or sending a child to camp, teach them to stay away from poison oak and poison ivy. These plans have an oily sap called urushiol that causes itchy rashes. Recognize poison ivy rashes by redness and itching, bumps and oozing blisters. Get some relief by using rose, lavender, and Roman chamomile essential oils. You can also use a diluted mixture of peppermint oil. The menthol in peppermint oil relieves the burning and itching that accompanies the rash. Drip several drops of essential oil into warm water. Soak a clean cloth in the water and wring it out. Apply this compress to the affected areas. Hopefully, the itching and pain will quickly stop.

Gallstones, formed by cholesterol that has crystallized from bile in the gallbladder, block the duct that comes from the gallbladder into the small intestine. Gallbladder attacks are very painful and can lead to infections or jaundice. Until you can see a doctor, use the healing power of essential oils. Grapefruit, geranium, rosemary, wintergreen and lime essential oils are suggestions. Dilute in a carrier oil at a ratio of 2 to 1 and apply 1-2 drops over the gallbladder area. You can also apply these essential oils as a warm compress.

Hiccups or the uncontrollable spasms of the diaphragm, caused by a sudden intake of breath and the closure of the glottis, can be debilitating. Something irritating the diaphragm or carbon dioxide in the bloodstream are possible causes of hiccups. They are annoying, can be painful and embarrassing. Get rid of hiccups by using sandalwood essential oil. Diffuse into the air or inhale directly from the bottle. Apply the oil to hands, tissues or on a cotton ball and inhale.

Shingles is a very nasty viral infection caused by the same virus that produces chickenpox. The virus is activated by stress or immune diseases. Symptoms include tingling, pain, and neuralgia and itching. Red blisters form and follow along nerve paths under the skin. Oils that give relief are melaleuca, eucalyptus, lavender, lemon geranium and bergamot. Mix ten drops of lavender, ten drops of melaleuca, and ten drops of thyme with one tablespoon of carrier oil. Apply on the bottoms of the feet. You can also apply 1-2 drops of any of these oils directly to the rash once you have blended them with a mild carrier oil.

Vertigo is a sensation that feels like the environment is moving or spinning. You may fall or feel nauseated. Ear infection, disorders or motion sickness can cause vertigo. Use ginger, helichrysum, geranium, basil and lavender to combat the symptoms of vertigo. Apply 1-2 drops of helichrysum, geranium, and lavender to the tops of each ear and massage it in. Apply the oils behind each ear, behind the jaw bone and just below the jaw. Apply 1-2 drops of basil behind and down each ear. You can do this multiple times a day until symptoms decrease.

Wound care requires a few key anti-microbial essential oils. Number one on the list is melaleuca or tea tree oil. With its properties as an antiseptic and antimicrobial it is perfect for cleaning and dressing wounds. You can also dip into your stores of lavender if you are treating a wound. Lavender speeds up the healing process of wounds and improves the formation of scar tissue. It is also pain-relieving. Use helichrysum to keep your wounds from turning septic. Helichrysum is safe to apply on wounds, cuts, and pricks or any other open sores that are in danger of becoming infected. Helichrysum is also a coagulant that helps with bleeding.

Essential oils can be used to ease the suffering of cancer patients. Essential oils are forms of supportive care and reduce anxiety and stress. Essential oils, massage and inhalation support and balance the mind, body and spirit. When combined with other complementary treatments, like massage therapy and acupuncture, symptoms of cancer can be managed.

Weight Loss

Were you aware that essential oils can help you lose weight? Although not endorsed by the Food and Drug Administration, personal and scientific profiles have highlighted the digestive and diuretic properties of grapefruit essential oil. Grapefruit has been proven to relieve fluid retention and help dissolve fat. Using massage, a therapist places a few drops of grapefruit essential oil into a carrier. Massaging into fatty areas of the body helps reduce cellulite. Smelling grapefruit essential oil also gives you a more energized feeling, and you may experience fewer hunger pangs.

Peppermint essential oil gives you a feeling of fullness. Dr. Alan Hirsch of the Smell and Taste Treatment and Research Institute of Chicago states that peppermint affects the part of the brain dealing hunger. Inhale peppermint essential oils throughout the day or just before each meal to curb your appetite.

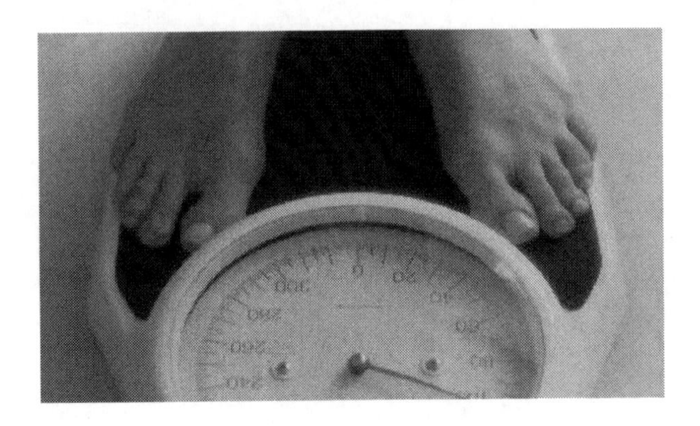

Weight Loss

Bergamot has a soothing effect on the mind and takes away your feelings of stress and hunger. Bergamot creates a sense of well-being. Combine bergamot with lavender to keep the stress away and avoid binge eating to calm down your stress.

Another citrus-based essential oil helping with weight loss is tangerine. This essential oil tones the skin and provides an agent to diminish the appearance of cellulite, stretch marks, and scars. Tangerine essential oil regulates metabolism and creates feelings of happiness. Do not go out in the sun after applying tangerine. Combine tangerine with bergamot or lavender for an extra feeling of wellness.

Rose geranium essential oil has mood-lifting qualities. These properties may just help you diminish your cellulite, reduce the effects of edema and fluid retention, and balance hormones. Rose geranium is one essential oil that has a GRAS rating from the FDA. This designation means rose geranium essential oil is recognized as safe to use.

First Aid Kit

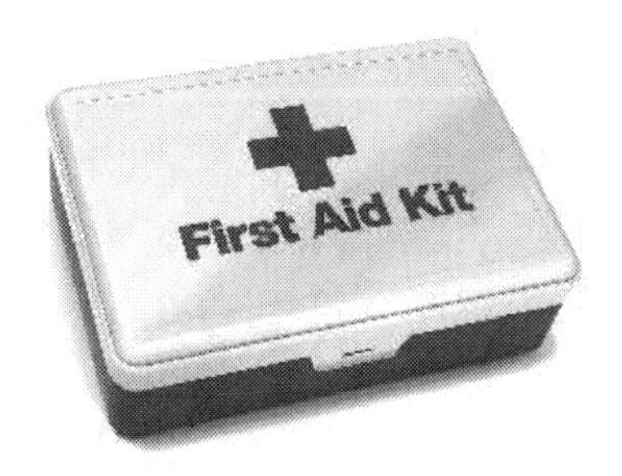

Assemble a first aid kit with these essential oils to help you with a variety of minor ailments and therapeutic uses. Essential oils have hundreds of benefits that you should take advantage of when a first aid kit is necessary. Essential oils are easy and convenient to use, and you can use the same products on your family and your pets. Multiple properties in essential oils make them perfect for a variety of uses.

Tea Tree oil refined from the Australian plant Melaleuca alterniflloria is topically and is perfect as that topical treatment. Tea tree essential oil is one of the best disinfectants in the essential oil tool box or first aid kit.

- One of the most versatile essential oils is lavender. It works on bruises, cuts and skin irritations. But it also relaxes your mind and reduces the levels of stress hormones in your blood. Lavender essential oil in a first aid kit helps with the emotional aspects of an emergency. You need to stay calm and keep your patient calm; lavender is the perfect solution.

Burns, cuts, stings and bruises will feel better if you apply one drop of lavender oil direct to the injury or sting site. Cover with a cool and damp cloths. Repeat compress application every 15 to 20 minutes. Apply until the pain goes away, or the damaged areas feel better.

- **Lavender essential oil** is also a first choice for minor burns and sunburns. It can be applied undiluted directly to the area or dilute if necessary. Lavender is known to soothe and help hydrate the skin. (If you have more severe burns, seek medical attention.)

- **Clove oil** should be in your first aid kit to help with toothaches. This essential oil has the largest antioxidant value of all the essential oils. It provides a great numbing effect and actually feels warm and soothing. You can put a drop or two of clove essential oil directly on the infected tooth.

- **Myrrh essential oil** has a warm and woody aroma used for skin and cleansing the body. Add a few drops to warm water to wash wounds. You can also rinse your mouth with warm war and a few drops of myrrh to promote healthy gums and get rid of mouth issues.

- **Peppermint oil** is a favorite of many people and not only for its smell but for stimulating the mind. Peppermint oil is known to intensify mental awareness. Dr. William N. Denver of the University of Cincinnati discovered that inhaling peppermint oil increased mental accuracy by almost 28%. You can also take **peppermint oil** internally. Mix a few drops in water and drink if you have indigestion.

- **Geranium essential oil** is a stress reliever when you have unruly patients. It is great for supporting the circulatory and nervous systems and does revitalize body tissues.

- **Lemon oil** can be used to detox the body and help with acne. A bit of lemon oil mixed 50/50 with a carrier will give you a burst of alertness, concentration and focus. Rub some lemon oil on pets. Fleas will run away!

- More **citrus oils include grapefruit**. It has properties quite similar to lemon oil. If you are fatigued or have jet lag, use grapefruit in a spray or a diffuser. Grapefruit is also a natural antiseptic. Add it to you homemade cleansers to keep your house free of germs.

- You have probably tried a bit of chamomile as a tea when you are feeling puckish. The essential oil of chamomile has relaxing properties. You can mix it with lavender or spray it on your pillow to find that pocket of sleep you need.

- **Frankincense** is very expensive but is also a must-have essential oil for your home. It can be used in a bath for relaxation and patted on bug bites. Frankincense has been used for thousands of years for depression, inflammation, immunity and to increase spiritual awareness. Thousands of years ago, frankincense was used a trading commodity.

- **Oregano** is a wonderful herb used in Italian and Mediterranean foods, and this essential oil is a flu fighter. Oregano has a strong taste and has natural antibacterial qualities. It fights colds and other flu-like sicknesses. You can take oregano internally. Put a few drops on your tongue and let it absorb into your body. The taste is different, but it works.

- **Eucalyptus essential oil** is great for cold sufferers. If you are congested, eucalyptus is your oil for relief. Eucalyptus is also used to relieve sore muscles. It has antibacterial properties and stimulates the immune system. Use eucalyptus essential oil in a vaporizer to loosen up mucus in a congested chest. You can also apply eucalyptus directing to the inside of your nose to relieve nasal congestion. Avoid actually ingesting eucalyptus or rubbing it on your skin in an undiluted form; it can be irritating.

- If you have plantar warts on your hands or feet and they are irritating, apply one drop of **oregano essential oil** to the wart then add one drop of lemon and one drop of peppermint. Cover the warts. Follow this recipe at least twice a day until the wart vanishes. If you have sensitive skin, dilute the oregano oil.
- If your children suffer from nightmares, make a spray that keeps the nightmares away. Mix five drops of **lavender oil** in one cup of distilled water. Mix in a fine-mist spray bottle. Let your child spray the monster away. If you are a grownup, and have nightmares, just spritz on your pillow. The monsters will go away for the night.

Mix five drops of lavender essential oil to three drops of tea tree essential oil, and add two drops of cypress essential oil. Add these oils to eight ounces of warm water to a spray bottle. Add in ½ teaspoon of salt and shake until the salt is dissolved. Use as a natural first aid spray.

Pet Care

You can use several different essential oils on your pets when you feel they are suffering. Dogs respond very well to essential oils, and these oils can be used safely for everything from fleas to ticks to bruises and bumps.

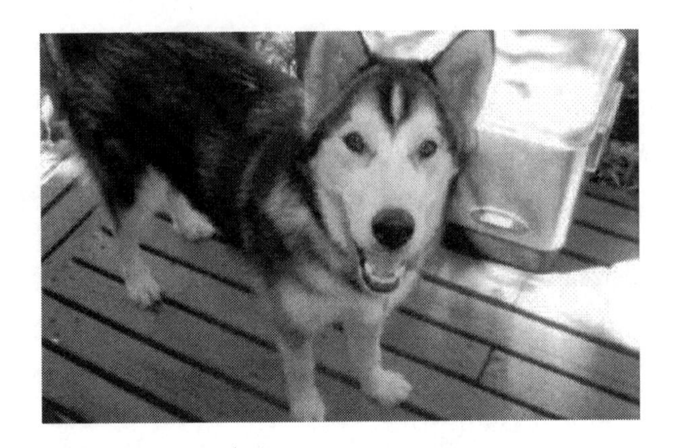

Essential oils are not toxic to your pet's body, they are easy to use, and perfect home remedies for dogs. Use essential oils to give your dog more concentration, focus, and anxiety as you train your dog. They do work.

Use therapeutic-grade essential oils for your pets. Perfume quality or aromatherapy grade oils will cause harm in your dogs. Therapeutic grade essential oils are steam distilled and do not contain any chemicals or additives.

- You can apply essential oils to dogs in several ways:
- Apply directly to the dog's skin,
- Place the oil in your palm and pet your dog from head to toe;
- Apply essential oils where the skin is thin, like the belly;
- Allow your dog to smell the essential oil from your hands or right out of the bottle.

If your dog is suffering from arthritis or osteoarthritis or rheumatoid arthritis, use wintergreen essential oil as a massage. Rub diluted wintergreen essential oils into paws or the belly. This is the best way to get the properties of wintergreen into the bloodstream. The most valuable property of wintergreen is its antispasmodic benefits.

You can also use tea tree essential oil that is known to help with arthritis in humans. Dilute the oil so it is not irritating and massage onto paws or the non-furry parts of the body–like the belly.

Keep a canine first aid kit with you when traveling with your dog. The best oils for this kit are lavender essential oil, peppermint, Frankincense and any ointments from a reputable dealer containing therapeutic grade essential oils.

Chapter 4

Holistic and Alternative Medicine

"This is the world's medicine, it's been there forever, we should take advantage of it".

—Dr. Oz

Holistic or alternative medicine is an approach to health and living that believes the causes of the problems must be found and dealt with within instead of simply treating the symptoms. Essential oils fit perfectly with alternative and holistic medicine; they are the natural way to soothe and heal symptoms.

Aromatherapy

The alternative medicine that uses essential oils is called aromatherapy.

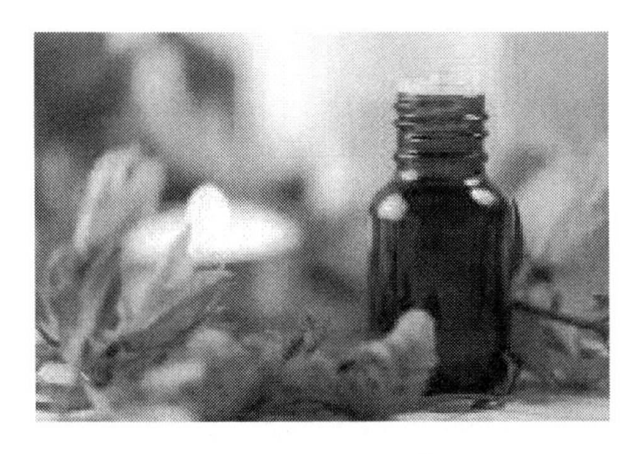

The Gift of Aromatherapy

Aromatherapy is the practice of using natural oils to enhance psychological and physical well-being. Inhaling essential oils is believed to stimulate brain functions. Oils can be absorbed through the skin and travel through the bloodstream to promote whole body health and wellness. Aromatherapists use blends of therapeutic essential oils in topical applications, massage, inhalation or water immersion to inspire a healing response in the body.

Practitioners of aromatherapy believe the fragrances in the oils stimulate nerves in the nose. These nerves send impulses to the part of the brain that controls memory and emotion. Depending on the oil, the results may be stimulating or calming. Aromatherapy works on the premise that oils interact with the body's hormones and enzymes to cause changes in pulse, blood pressure, and emotion. It is also a theory that fragrance of certain oils stimulates the body to fight pain.

Aromatherapy promotes relaxation and helps relieve stress and depression. It is not positively known if aromatherapy using essential oils cures illnesses, but it does make them livable.

Aromatherapy is safe at the hands of an expert. Massage therapists, nurses, and counselors have been taught how to use essential oils, and they can understand how to augment traditional medicine with alternative medicine to create a whole healing package.

Aromatherapists use essential oil on the skin, or as dermal applications, diffused, inhaled, or ingested. Every one of these methods has safety issues that need to be taken into consideration. Oils that are rich in aldehydes and phenols can cause skin reactions. Essential oils that have these constituents must always be diluted prior to application to the skin. Aromatherapists blend these essential oils with other essential oils and gentle carriers to mitigate their irritant effects.

When using oils on the skin in massage therapy, dilutions are done between 1 and 5 percent. It is also advised to try a bit of essential oil in a carrier on a very small and inconspicuous area spot before using it all over your body.

Ayurveda

Practitioners of Ayurveda use essential oils almost reverently. Ayurvedic medicine is a system of Hindu traditional medicine used for over thousands of years. Ayurveda is native to the Indian continent but is making its way to western cultures. Ayurveda makes use of aromatherapy in many of its practices, and essential oils are used to enhanced the sense of smell and contribute to physical and mental health. Essential oils, according to the Ayurveda system, allows the body to fight against illnesses by bringing balance to the entire system. Ayurveda does not promote taking essential oils internally; in fact Ayurveda practitioners frown on the practice of some holistic practitioners who urge ingesting essential oils to heal illnesses.

It is an Ayurveda belief that it is difficult to control the internal dosages of essential oils. The high volatility of the plant oils will damage tissues, systems or functions rather than heal them if taken internally. Ayurveda prefers to use essential oils in aromatherapy and inhalation therapies.

Acupuncture

Acupuncture is an alternative medicine treatment that has been used in Chinese medicine for over 5,000 years. It literally means piercing, and fine needs are inserted at specific acupoints on the body. The stimulation of these points redistributes the flow of energy to restore health.

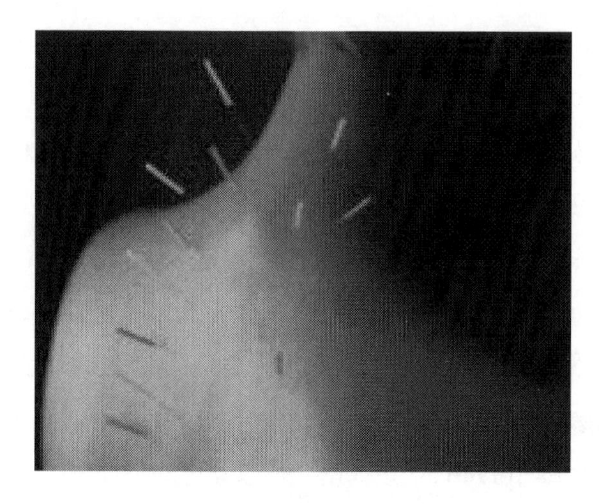

Acupuncture for Back Pain

Acupuncture treatment offers similar beneficial properties to essential oils. Acupuncturists use the healing properties of pure essential oils to increase health and well-being. Essential oils are used not just for inhalation and massage, but on the acupuncture needles themselves. Dipping the acupuncture needles in an essential oil increases the benefit of the acupuncture retreatment. Using essential oils with acupuncture is labeled as medicated needle acupuncture.

Japanese Palpitation/Acupuncture

Japanese acupuncture includes many different styles of Chinese acupuncture, but refined in Japan. Japanese acupuncture uses palpitation at every acupuncture point before treating with the needles. Japanese acupuncture uses extremely thin needles and shallow insertion versus thicker needles and deep insertion used by Chinese acupuncture. Japanese acupuncture also uses moxibustion or warming acupoints by burning moxa, a substance derived from the mugwort plant.

One system of healing, Body-Feedback™ created by Michelle Buchanan, uses the Japanese acupuncture techniques of palpation, warming acupoints and inhalation therapies. Inhaling essential oils produces a temporary response in the brain, and these responses are measured by palpating specific areas of the body to locate body disturbances.

The founder feels that the effectiveness of therapeutic-grade essential oils is enhanced by combining them with the ancient acupuncture palpation method. The method determines which essential oils resonate with your body through a series of palpation and inhalation techniques. The theory is designed around essential oils easily penetrating your skin, muscle, fat and connective tissues and allowing rapid absorption into the bloodstream to promote healing.

Furthermore, the premise is essential oils, therapeutic-grade, have high electrical frequencies and hold great healing potential. In other words, if you are sick or injured you will feel well within minutes when the right essential oils are administered in the right way. One way this is established, the founder believes, is through Japanese palpitation and acupuncture.

Chapter 5

Home and Personal Use

"I have spent the last two day striving to write a concise easy guide to essential oils and their safety and it ended up being just an enormous dump of information."

—Crunchy Betty

It is impossible to get rid of every germ in your home, but with essential oils you have a fighting chance. Germs pass freely from a surface to another surface that makes every surface in your home a positive Petri dish. Read the labels of mainstream home products, and you will find a list of toxic ingredients that research shows are harmful in every way. It would be good to stop using harmful cleaners.

Essential oils are safe alternatives for the harsh products you use every day. Use natural and green ways to make your own cleaning and personal care products and use essential oils to get an added boost.

Personal Use

Essential oils are used in personal care products and cosmetics because of their nourishing benefits and unique scents. They are also renowned for enhancing complexions and promoting general health of skin and hair. There are recipes for keeping hair smooth and shiny listed in ancient Egyptian papyrus scrolls. Once these recipes were translated, they became a staple of personal care. The current trend toward products that are "green" has prompted many people to look into essential oils for everyday personal care products. Essential oils are perfect for adding to your shampoos, conditions, moisturizers, skin cleansers, and toothpastes. Specific essential oils promote hair and body health by stimulating circulation, relieving pain, improving flexibility, and improving everyday living.

Shampoos and Conditioners

Chamomile shampoo and or conditioners are very soothing. They retract skin cells that have become inflamed from chemical procedures and help to relieve scaly and itchy scalps.

Lavender is awesome and soothes the scalp and the hair. Lavender in baby shampoo is very helpful in calming infants.

Lemon gives golden highlights to blond hair. It works well as a treatment for dry hair, dandruff, lice and active sebaceous glands.

Be cautious when using lemon essential oil; too much lemon in your hair may dry out hair strands and cause an itchy scalp.

Tea tree essential oil has been used in shampoos and conditioners for years. Tea tree works to clear up scalp conditions like dandruff and psoriasis that cause inflammation or dryness. Tea tree essential oil can be combined with jojoba oil to deep-cleanse the scalp.

Thyme essential oils are also remarkable for hair. Thyme is used to provide shine and absolute cleanliness and works well when used with very mild cleansing agents. Combine thyme with ylang-ylang to effectively clean your hair.

Cosmetics

Consumers look for cosmetics and beauty products that are more than pretty shades or scented moisturizers. Popular cosmetics are those that improve skin, are relaxing, and considered green and safe. According to researchers, "We have the pioneers of aromatherapy to thank for [ethical shopping.]" Essential oils are used in beauty products for their therapeutic properties. Major cosmetic brands include essential oils in their formulas to give an added punch to their cosmetic lines. Essential oils are used in cosmetics to help with skin issues or allergic reactions to cosmetic formulas. These types of cosmetics may be expensive, and that is okay. You can find cosmetic products containing essential oils marketed as aromatherapy cosmetics. The benefits of essential oils in cosmetics are the aromas that make the cosmetics pleasant-smelling and skin-enhancing.

Essential oils or aromatherapy oils are highly concentrated and use the volatile essences of plants. Using essential oils in cosmetics can have the added benefit of providing calming or stimulating properties. Essential oils added to natural cosmetics will beautify the skin and body, stimulate the senses, and provide confidence you are using pure products.

Studies from the Netherlands have shown that consumers love the earthy, woodsy, and fresh scents that come from 100% pure essential oils in their cosmetics. No other synthetic additives provide this same scent and feeling of well-being. Consumers are rapidly realizing that if you want purity, rich smell, and environmentally friendly cosmetics, essential oils needs to be a listed ingredient.

Essential oils suppliers are becoming aware of their part in the increasingly environmentally friendly cosmetic industry. Ethical essential oil distillers are ramping up efforts to protect pure oils from being turned into derivatives and manufactured into substandard cosmetics.

Essential oils are perfect for facial moisturizers, lotions, and refreshers. One excellent natural moisturizer recipe uses ten drops of carrot seed essential oil, six drops of myrrh essential oil, four drops of lavender, four drops of frankincense, and a carrier oil of coconut oil. Whip all ingredients with a mixer until fluffy and light. Store in a glass jar. You will be amazed at the wonderful moisturizing properties of this do-it-yourself essential moisturizing cream.

Do you want radiant skin? Use essentials oils in 1/2 teaspoon of almond oil. Add 1/3 cup of castile soap plus ten drops of ylang-ylang essential oil. Mix in six drops of patchouli essential oil, four drops of lemongrass essential oil and 2/3 cups of filtered water. Swirl everything together to combine. Fill a container with filtered water and keep on your bathroom vanity whenever you need to cleanse or refresh your face.

Make toothpaste using essential oils for a healthier and brighter smile:

5 parts Calcium powder

1 part Diatomaceous Earth

2 parts Baking Soda

3 parts Xylitol Powder

3-5 part coconut oil for texture

Mint, cinnamon, orange essential oils for taste

Mix all ingredients together, preferably in a food blender, and store in a small container.

Natural Cleaning

Conventional cleaners are formulated with harsh chemicals that damage the environment. There are safe, effective alternatives that are easy to make and safe to use. Many of these natural and homemade cleaners utilize essential oils for higher protection and cleaning power. The most popular essential oils for cleaning include the following herbs.

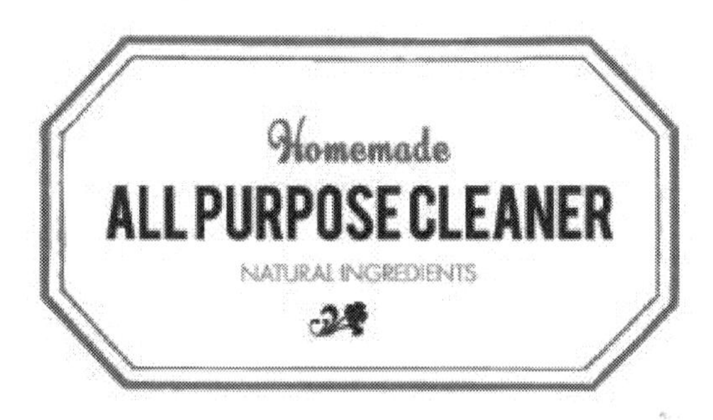

Basil essential oil is an anti-infectious and antibacterial oil. It can be used topically without with dilution, used in cooking or taken internally via capsules. Dilute it in water with lemon oil to keep kitchen surfaces germ-free and smelling awesome.

Chamomile essential oil has a scent of fruit and herbs and is known to be soothing and calming. The scent is amazing and blends well with florals, citruses, and lemon essential oils. Add several drops of chamomile to warm water or add directly to liquid laundry detergents.

Cinnamon essential oil has a spicy and sweet scent and blends well with orange or tangerine. It makes a room smell almost

"Christmasy." Cinnamon should not be used alone in homemade cleaners but just add a few drops to bring in a warming touch. Cinnamon works well as a room deodorizer in either spray form or a diffuser.

Geranium essential oil is a floral scent, smells a bit like roses, and is somewhat pungent. Often geranium essential oils blend with rose essential oil to make a floral scent for laundry supplies. Geranium oil also combines well with lavender, rosemary, orange, and lemon. Just image how wonderful your linens will smell with the addition of any essential oil. You can also use a combination of geranium and lemon essential oils in dish water to clean your dishes.

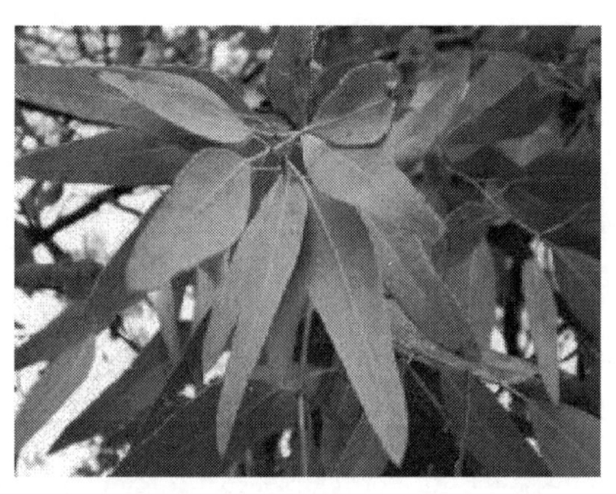

Eucalyptus plant

Eucalyptus essential oils have a sharp and very pungent odor. Eucalyptus almost smells like camphor combined with a woodsy scent. Eucalyptus oils mix well with pine, rosemary, and tea tree oils. Lavender and lemon are also compatible with eucalyptus essential oils and when used in warm water are great for disinfecting a sick room.

Jojoba essential oil added to any natural polisher will give your furniture shine without harmful additives. You can make your own natural wood cleaner by mixing ¼ cup white vinegar with lemon essential oil and a tablespoon of olive oil. Use this in a spray bottle or put a small amount on a rag and dust away.

Try lavender with its clean, floral and fresh scent to soothe, calm and relax your home environment. Lavender is one of the most popular essential oils for cleaning. It blends well with most other essential oils and is especially effective when combined with citrus essential oils.

Lemon essential oil is wonderful and has a clean and fresh scent. It is associated with house cleaning and fresh smells. It is the most common scent used in household cleaners and is awesome at cutting kitchen grease. Add lemon essential oil to warm water with vinegar and spray away to keep germs off your drain boards.

Lemon and lime essential oils added to warm water in a spray bottle will help remove stickers, crayons, and other marks from paint.

Peppermint essential oils are wonderful for keeping your home smelling minty fresh. Peppermint blends well with other popular essential oils. Use peppermint as a natural pest deterrent, room deodorizer, and cleaning oil.

Rose essential oil is perfect for cleaning and adding to laundry supplies like fabric softeners and laundry detergents. Rose essential oil is somewhat expensive since it takes thousands of rose petals to create a bottle of essential oil, so use it sparingly. Rose oil is often combined with geranium oil to create a less expensive but similar scent. Drop two or three drops in your washer as it is agitating. You will be amazed at the smell of your laundry.

Pine essential oil is a common scent used for cleaning products. It has antimicrobial properties and acts as deodorizer. It blends well with lemon, lavender, and eucalyptus. Use in a spray bottle or dip your rag in a solution of warm water, pine, lemon, and lavender. Your home will soon be germ-free.

Tea tree essential oil is useful for cleaning and it has antiseptic, antimicrobial and antifungal properties. The scent is spicy yet warm and has a camphor undertone. If you don't care for the fragrance of tea tree oil, blend it with other essential oils to improve the fragrance. Tea Tree essential oils are one of the three most indispensable oils to keep in your home for cleaning. (The other two are lavender and lemon essential oils).

Some very nice blends for homemade all-purpose cleaners use citrus essential oils, lemon, lime or grapefruit, because of their great fragrances and their degreasing properties. For a very effective and great smelling degreaser and germ killer, use the following recipe:

Combine the following ingredients in a spray bottle with warm water:

- Four parts lime essential oil
- Two parts sweet orange essential oil
- One part grapefruit essential oil.
- Spray away for a cleaner home.
- Cleaning your floors can be more powerful by adding:
- Two parts pine essential oil
- One part cypress essential oil.

Blend in warm water and mop away!

Natural carpet deodorizers and scented scrubbers are easy to make.

Combine essential oils with baking soda:

Two parts lavender essential oil,

One part vanilla essential oil

Mix with one 16 oz. box of baking soda. Sprinkle on your carpets as need for odor control. You can also use this same formula for scrubbing counters, sinks, bathtubs and other hard surfaces.

Keep your children's rooms clean and as germ-free as you can by using a mixture of antiviral essential oil blends in water. Several drops of the best antiviral essential oils to a spray bottle of warm water and vinegar will do wonders to get rid of cold and flu germs and those nasty germy smells. Germ killing essential oils include bergamot, rosemary, lavender, lemon, tea tree, and eucalyptus.

Formulate your own germ-destroying spray for traveling. Mix essential oils (any of them will work) in a one ounce bottle with a spray cap. Shake to blend and take with you on a plane. You can mist yourself and your seat using this mixture. Use in your hotel room and rental car to keep other people's germs at bay.

Healthy Cooking

Used sparingly, natural essential oils add intense flavor and aroma to just about anything you cook. Essential oils are great in candies, chocolates, frostings, soups and marinades. These wonderful highly concentrated, volatile essences of plants will add a natural blend to your cooking. Peppermint, lemon and orange are used to flavor desserts. Thyme and marjoram are delightful for flavoring savory foods such as stews and sauces. Lavender and bergamot oils are popular in chocolate crafting.

Use essential oils in place of spices. Substitute lemon essential oil for lemon zest and orange oil for orange zest. No more grating and scrubbing your knuckles!

Add variety and flavor to your cooking. Move over spices in your spice cabinet and add essential oils. They have rich aromas that add a delicious kick of flavor to recipes. Add a drop or two of lime to fresh salsa or your favorite Italian-inspired marinade. Drop a bit of lemon on grilled fish, peppermint essential oil to hot cocoa, basil and oregano to homemade pasta sauces.

Just a drop replaces a teaspoon of dried herbs or spices. For essential oils such as thyme, oregano, marjoram and rosemary stir in one drop to your foods as you serve the dish. Oils with robust flavors can be cooked in soups and stews to produce an awesome flavor. The best way to use essential oils in cooking is to start small and add more as needed.

The paramount essential oils for cooking include anise, bergamot, caraway, chamomile, clove, eucalyptus, ginger, grapefruit and juniper berry. Add lavender, lemon, lime marjoram, nutmeg, orange and oregano to your dishes as per your taste. Oregano is perfect in Italian dishes and peppermint is lovely in chocolate recipes. Tangerine, thyme, and wintergreen are also popular cooking essential oils.

Insect Repellents

Natural insect repellents can be made with several types of essential oils. Most oils keep bugs away and prevent bites and stings. Natural insect repellents are much better than synthetic and chemical based repellents. Commercial insect repellents have toxic effects on humans and the environment.

There are studies proving that eucalyptus essential oil is very offensive to mosquitoes. One species of eucalyptus, lemon eucalyptus essential oil, is almost comparable to products that use low levels of DEET or diethyltoluamide. DEET was developed by the United States Army to keep bugs away during jungle warfare during WWII. DEET is an irritant and can cause severe epidermal reactions. Eucalyptus essential oil will not damage your skin when combined with a carrier and sprayed.

Citronella essential oil has active compounds that are high in repellent activity. Burning citronella-based candles ward off sand flies and mosquitoes.

In a study of 38 different essential oils, researchers found clove oil offered the highest protection against mosquito species than any other essential oils. Patchouli essential oil provides almost two hours of complete repellency and is almost as effective as clove essential oil.

Essential oils are very potent. Take caution when making use of any essential oil as a natural insect repellent. Blend your essential oils with a carrier oil such as avocado, sweet almond or jojoba. Avoid applying natural insect repellents directly to your skin.

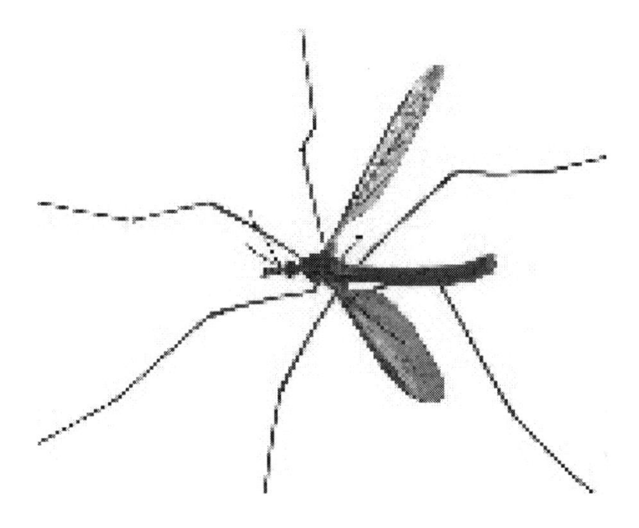

Mosquito

Chapter 6

Properties of Popular Essential Oils

"Aromatherapy may promote relaxation and help relieve stress. It has also been used to help treat a wide range of physical and mental conditions."

—Web MD

Essential oils are highly concentrated and you only need a drop or two. Due to their powerful antioxidant properties, essential oils have been used for thousands of years in soaps, perfumes, aromatherapy, and skin care products as well as for medical purposes. The healing value within essential oils is remarkable and there are a number of different health and emotional concerns that can be calmed. Arthritis, sore throats, congestion, digestive issues, joint pains, muscle fatigue, stress and anger are just a few of those concerns.

There are hundreds of essential oils and blends with their own unique powers and health benefits. Learning the ones that are effective in treating your condition takes research, study and experimentation. Also remember to follow directions before you actually use essential oils.

You medicine cabinet should hold these essential oils:

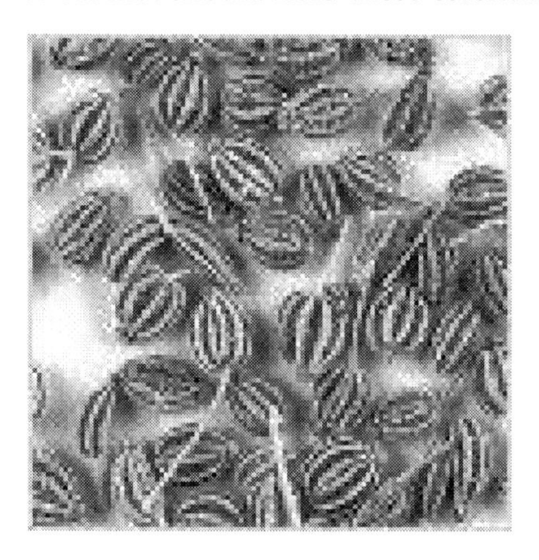

Ajowan essential oils have a woody and spicy fragrance; they almost smell like thyme. Flowers and seeds are steam distilled to extract the essential oil from ajowan. Ajowan essential oil is considered a "hot" oil and a carrier must be used when applying to the skin. According to Ayurveda, ajowan essential oil used correctly brings up angry feelings and allows these feeling to clear.

- Basil essential oil is a nerve tonic and used for sharpening memories. It is also a great when used to get rid of phlegm from bronchial tubes. Indigestion, constipation and nausea can be controlled by using basil. The leaves and seeds of the basil plant are the medicinal part of this herb. Basil is used topically and massaged into the skin. Steam distil basil leaves for the essential oils.

- Bergamot is a citrus-scented essential oil. In an impure form bergamot is used in colognes and perfumes. Take a whiff of bergamot and your stress and anxiety might just blow away. Use bergamot if you suffer from eczema. Dilute bergamot in a carrier oil before you apply to the skin. It can burn skin. Bergamot is taken out of Citrus aurantium var bergamia trees native to South East Asia. It can also be found in Europe, Italy and along the Ivory Coast. Its scent is fresh smelling, and the oil is great for generating a happy feeling, getting rid of urinary tract infections and boosting the liver. It also fights acne, oily skin and eczema and cold sores.

- Birch essential oil is a tonic, disinfectant, stimulant and antidepressant. It detoxifies your body and is wonderful when used as an antiseptic. There are two types of birch, the White Birch or Silver Birch. Birch has been used as a decorative tree and a medicinal plant since ancient times.

- Black pepper essential oil is known as a digestive, diaphoretic, and antispasmodic substance. Black pepper is the dried fruit of the pepper plant and is known as a culinary spice. Thousands of years ago pepper was traded for gold and was one of the most valued items exported from India. Black pepper is a digestive aid and is beneficial since it stimulates the entire digestive system from the glands in the mouth to the large intestine. Usually black pepper is used as an ingested essential oil.

- Carrot seed essential oil is used in aromatherapy and as an antiseptic, disinfectant, anticarcinogenic and diuretic substance. It is extracted via steam distillation from the dried seeds of wild carrots and from the plant itself. It is common in Europe and often known as Queen Anne's Lace. If you want to retain your youth and look young, carrot seed essential oils stop free radicals from doing harm to your tissues. It protects skin from wrinkles, keeps hair from turning white, and joints from stiffening. This very powerful essential oil is a virtual fountain of youth.

- Cassia essential oil comes from the laurel bush. Bark is steam distilled for its antibacterial and antifungal properties. Medicinally, cassia is used for colds and flu symptoms plus colic and diarrhea. It provides powerful support to different essential blends when used in small quantities. Be careful with cassia essential oil. When used in large doses it can result in sensitivity. Cassia is known as Chinese Cinnamon and has been used for medicinal purposes for thousands of years.

- Chamomile is one of the most powerful calming essential oils. It is a mood booster. You can use Chamomile in steam, vapor therapies, sprays and massage oils to relieve stress. Chamomile comes from the flowers of the

Chamomile plant and these little flowers look almost like daisies. Roman Chamomile is more calming and works as a sedative. German chamomile is anti-inflammatory due to Azulene, a compound found it its flowers. A wonderful cup of chamomile tea with a drop of chamomile essential oil is very effective in fighting depression and eliminating feelings of sadness and disappointment.

- Cinnamon originated in tropical Asia and is a very popular spice and cuisine enhancer. The shrub grows in almost every tropical region of the world. It has vast medicinal properties and has a prominent position in traditional medicines and in Ayurveda, an Indian alternative medicine. Cinnamon essential oil boosts the activity of the brain and helps to remove nervous tension and memory loss. Cinnamon essential oils can support removal of blood impurities and has the ability to control blood sugar. Diabetics find cinnamon a great aid in lowering blood sugar and regulating insulin use.

- Clary Sage essential oil is known for its health benefits as an antidepressant, anticonvulsive, and antispasmodic oil. It comes from the buds and leaves of the Clary Sage plant or Salvia Sclarea. It is really an herb originally native to Europe. It has awesome properties and has been used as a preparation for vision and eye health. Clary sage in a spray bottle or a diffuser is a soft aphrodisiac. Use clary sage as an antiseptic for wounds to prevent tetanus germs.

Keep a bottle of this essential in your collection to help boost self-esteem, confidence and hope.

- Clove oil has been used for centuries for dental issues. It lessens toothaches, cold sores, gum issues and canker sores. It is very strong and must be diluted if you have sensitive teeth, gums or skin; otherwise you can place a drop of clove oil directly on the infected tooth. It can also cure athlete's foot, insect bites, bruises, and ear aches. Add clove oil to a diffuser in your home to keep mosquitoes away. Clove essential oil comes from an evergreen tree that produces a flower called a clove bud. The oil is highly prized for its diabetic properties and helps control blood sugar levels. The phenol concentration in clove essential oil is one of the highest in spice plants.

- Coriander essential oils come from seeds are steam distilled. Coriander is an analgesic, antibacterial, and antifungal essential oil. It has sedative and anti-inflammatory properties. It is used to fight digestive spasms and anorexia. Coriander can regulate pain. It does have aphrodisiac properties.

- Eucalyptus essential oil comes from Australia and has a very recognizable and strong scent. Eucalyptus essential oil is used to treat chest congestion, asthma attacks, and has been used to stifle the pain of fibromyalgia. It has very high disinfectant properties, and can be sprayed around your kitchen and bathroom to help eliminate germs and odors.

- Frankincense essential oil is a must have in any essential oil collection. It is perfect for treating acne, warts, cysts and insect bites. It is a very good disinfectant. It also helps relieve stress, is used to get rid of migraines. Frankincense comes from a tree that exudes a milky white sap. Boswellia trees, the source of frankincense oil, grows in Africa, Yemen, Oman, Somalia and Ethiopia. Oman has traded frankincense essential oil for thousands of years and this oil is very valuable. Frankincense has a woody, spicy, earthy and slightly fruity aroma. It is calming and relaxing and a bit more expensive than other essential oils.

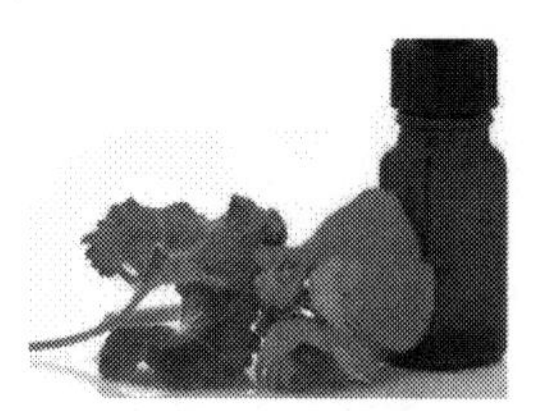

Geranium essential oil

- Geranium essential oil comes from the steam distillation of the leaves. It has a very strong aroma and is used for cellulites, dull skin, lice, oily skin, and acne. The main function of geranium essential oil is as an astringent. It is also antibacterial and antimicrobial and helps keep you safe from developing infections.

- Ginger essential oil increases circulation and when blended with lemon essential oil it is doubly effective. Ginger essential oil is a great digestive aid and is used by arthritis sufferers when blended with juniper essential oil. Ginger tea with several drops of ginger essential oil will help in the treatment of nausea and morning sickness. Ginger essential oil comes from the rhizomes or the roots of the ginger plant. West African women weave belts of ginger to bring back their partners and awaken their sexual interest. This attribute has probably not been highly advertised in Western Cultures. Ginger is very safe for stomach disorders in people and in pets. Place a drop on your dog's paw if they are feeling ill.

- Grapefruit essential oil is best when used to brighten up your skin. This oil in a carrier oil will stimulate the lymphatic system and is also a diuretic. It is known to treat obesity and there are grapefruit diets available all over the internet. If you need an essential oil to cut through the sluggishness of your mind during certain times of the day, inhale grapefruit oil. You will find it very refreshing. Grapefruit essential oil comes from cold-pressing the peel. Use grapefruit oils as an antioxidant, disinfectant, stimulant and antiseptic.

- Juniper essential oil is the perfect antiseptic, sudorific, diuretic, antispasmodic and astringent agent. The oils are obtained through steam distillation of all parts of the tree–the needles, powered fruit and wood. Juniper is an evergreen shrub grown in Europe and North America. It smells wonderful and has very remarkable health benefits. Those wounded in wars or sporting events years ago were treated with juniper essential oil. Use it to protect wounds from developing tetanus.

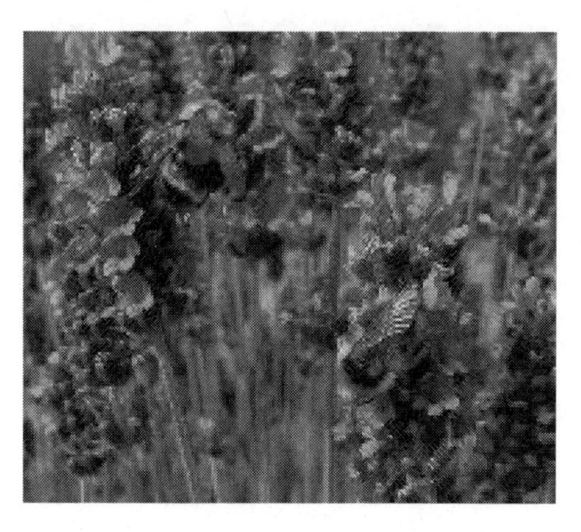

Lavender being pollinated

Lavender is one of the most versatile oils and is used for its comforting properties. Lavender diminishes stress in the mind and body, reduces inflammation and is also a stress reducer. Apply this oil to a minor area of your skin or add one or two drops to a diffuser. It is also nice on a pillow to give you a good night's sleep. When an elderly patient in a home-care situation became particularly agitated, lavender sprayed into her room and on her pillow was very calming. It also helped the care-taker calm down.

- Lemon oil has amazing benefits. You can use it to polish furniture or add to laundry soap, spray cleaners or floor cleaners. You can use lemon essential oil to stop bad breath just by putting a few drops in a glass and gargling. Lemon essential oil comes from the peel of the lemon, and is the most popular citrus fruit in the world. Health benefits of lemon essential oil come from its stimulating and anti-infection properties. It is also a detoxifying, antiseptic, disinfectant and helps to treat stress disorders fevers, and infections. Blend lemon essential oils with ylang-ylang essential oil, tea tree, geranium or sandalwood for a wonderful and relaxing massage.

- Marjoram essential oil comes from the mint family. It is steam distilled form the leaves and is used as an antibacterial and anti-infectious oil. It is known as a diuretic, expectorant and tonic. Marjoram essential oil has been used for hundreds of years as an analgesic, antispasmodic, and to control sexual desires or as an aphrodisiac.

- Melissa or lemon balm is also a member of the mint family. It is distilled by steaming the leaves. Used as an antihistamine, hypertensive, and nervine sedative, Melissa is also antibacterial. Clean up your cold sores by applying Melissa preparations to the sore. Melissa essential oil is used in many different types of balms because of its soothing properties. It does have a sweet and very pleasant aroma.

- Myrrh essential oil comes from the resin of its parent plant and is native to Egypt. Myrrh has antimicrobial, astringent, expectorant, and antifungal properties. When used properly myrrh does not allow microbes to grow or infect your system. It is great for fevers, food poisoning, coughs and colds. It helps to clean out wounds and keeps them from being infected. Do be careful when using myrrh essential oil. It does have toxic effects if used in excess.
- Neem essential is an organic oil from India. It is a very versatile restorative oil and used in alternative medicines. The neem seed is organically grown in the coastal Indian state of Tamil Nadu. It is a detoxifying agent and is awesome for keeping the hair and scalp clear. It is also used as an oil with other oils to keep the teeth and gums clean.

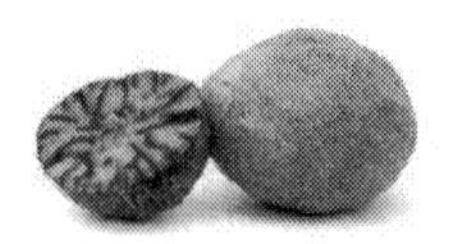

Nutmeg fruit

Nutmeg essential oil has a remarkable ability to treat stress, pain and heart disorders. You can fight bad breath and cough with nutmeg essential oil. Use it as a sedative and for its relaxing and anti-inflammatory properties. The nutmeg tree grows up to 70 feet tall and the oil is obtained from the seed of the nutmeg tree fruit. Nutmeg oil was once believed to be effective against the plague and was a popular oil during the Elizabethan era.

- Orange essential oils are perfect as anti-inflammatory, antidepressants, antispasmodics and as sedatives. The essential oil is obtained from the peels of oranges via cold compression. Orange essential oil is a mild aphrodisiac and aromatherapists claim that regular use of orange oil can cure frigidity, erectile problems, and loss of interest in sex. This oil also provides quick and effective relief from inflammations.

- Oregano essential oil is an antiviral, antibacterial, antifungal, anti-parasitic, and an antioxidant. Oregano is also an expectorant and loosens up mucus and phlegm in the respiratory tracts. It was first used in ancient Greece to treat bacterial infections on the skin or in wounds. Oregano means "delight of the mountains" and the oils are distracted through steam distillation of fresh oregano leaves. Oregano is traditionally used in one of three ways; aromatically, topically on the skin or through a carrier oil.

- Patchouli essential oil is used as an antidepressant, body toner, and antiseptic. It is highly sought after as an aphrodisiac, an astringent, and is used to drive away disappointment and tension. This oil has high insect repellant properties, and patchouli is one of the most versatile of the essential oils. Beware of using too many drops of this oil in any mixtures or alone. It has a strong scent and many people do not care for the aroma.

- Peppermint is awesome and provides you with a burst of energy. Your mental alertness will be improved, and peppermint just makes you feel good. Use it as a massage oil, lotion, or mouthwash. You can also add peppermint to steaming water to calm down symptoms of congestion. Add a drop of peppermint oil to your herbal tea. Your digestion will be greatly improved.

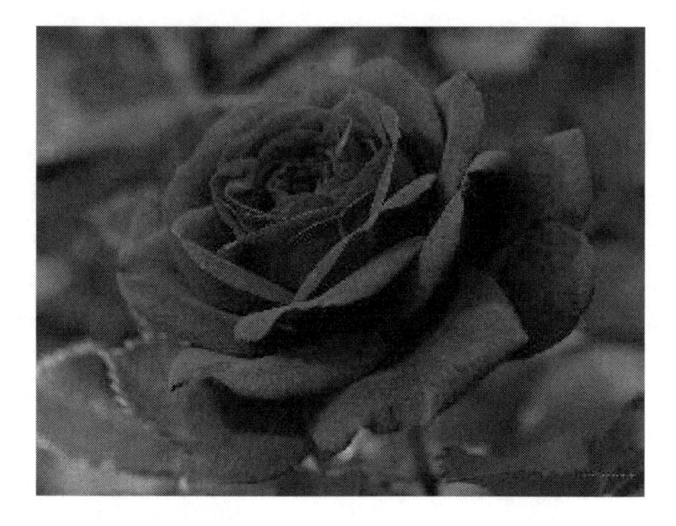

Rose

- Roses are considered the most beautiful flower in the world and the flower is the integral part of rose essential oil. Rose essential oils contribute to your psychological health. Rose oil is an antidepressant and increases self-esteem, mental strength, and confidence. Rose oil fights depression and is always used in aromatherapy as a massage oil. It arouses positive thoughts, feelings of hope and spiritual relaxation. Rose essential oil sis awesome and romantic when added to a diffuser.

- Rosemary essential oil has awesome rejuvenating effects. Use rosemary to relieve headaches, boost memory, stop stress from overtaking your life and stimulate circulation in the scalp. Add a bit of rosemary essential oil to your shampoo and have healthy and shiny hair. Rosemary essential oil is also great for detoxifying the liver and helping to release bile. Grab rosemary oil and infuse it when you are studying. It is an excellent nerve tonic and brain stimulator. It helps increase concentration and supports you when studying. Whenever your brain feels tired, inhale a bit of rosemary essential oil. It will remove your boredom and renew mental energy.

- Sandalwood helps calm and focus your senses. Drop in a couple of drops of sandalwood essential oil into your body lotion. Your skin will be hydrated and your tension relieved. Sandalwood comes from an evergreen tree native to southern Asia. The essential oil comes from the heartwood of the tree. Sandalwood is awesome as an antidepressant, antiviral, immune stimulant, calming, astringent, and antiseptic. If you are having a hard time sleeping, sandalwood encourages deep relaxation. An interesting note, sandalwood was used to embalm the dead in ancient Egypt and was used in soul-releasing ceremonies.

- Tea Tree essential oil is a must have in your essential collection. It is one of the most popular and effective essential oils. The oil is made from the leaves of the plant Melaleuca alterniflоria and is native to Australia. Tea tree essential oil is awesome for helping cure acne, fungal infections of the nails, and athlete's foot. Mixing tea-tree oil with a little silver helps clear up infected skin wounds.
- Vetiver essential oil comes from grasses. It is steam distilled from the roots which releases its mild, earthy and somewhat musky smell. Vetiver has a cooling effect on the body and the mind. Vetiver is not as well-known as most other essential oils but it is great for calming down a restless person, can be used as a sedative and is used as an antispasmodic. Vetiver grows all over the Indian subcontinent and the plant itself is used in cooling, foods and beverages.
- Wintergreen essential oil or oil of wintergreen is an essential oil that is highly sought after by people who are suffering from rheumatism, gout and pain in their joints and bones. The leaves are steam distilled and the analgesic properties of wintergreen are awesome. It is also a great antiseptic, disinfectant and bone stimulant. Wintergreen smells amazing and the scent is warming. In Colonial America, Indians and settlers used wintergreen as a tea.

- White fir comes from the conifer and it needles are steam distilled. White fir is analgesic, anti-arthritic, and is a great expectorant. Use a couple of drops in warm water and drink when you need to clear out your respiratory system. It is also great as a steam inhalant or used as a spray. Use as a massage oil to help with respiratory issues and increase energy stores.

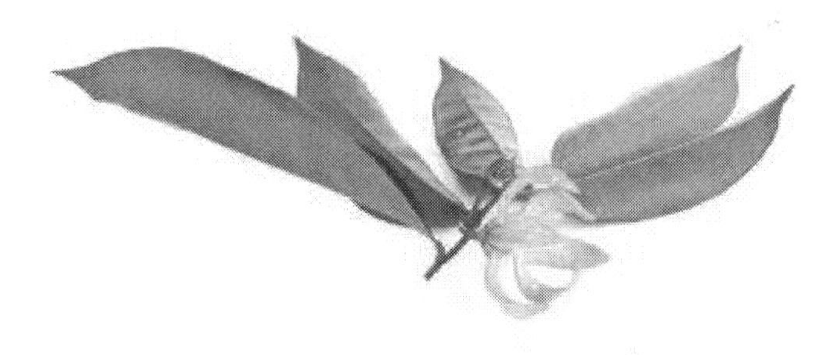

Ylang-Ylang

Ylang-ylang comes from a tropical tree native to Asia and is scientifically called Cananga odorata. The flowers are used to reduce heart palpitations and blood pressure. You may also find this jasmine-like scent used as an aphrodisiac. Just add a few drops of ylang-ylang oil in a hot bath and melt the days' stresses away. The scent can be overpowering if you are sensitive to heavy floral scents.

There many ways essential oils can be blended together to contribute to health and well-being. Study, research and experiment.

Chapter 7

Recipes for Using Essential Oils

"Have you ever wanted to make our own aromatherapy essential oil recipes? Maybe you've dabbled in aromatherapy before or perhaps you are a newcomer."

—*Essential Oil Recipes*

Essential oils can be used in everyday life to improve your health as well as your emotional and mental well-being. Easy aromatherapy recipes for beginners include simple tried and true ways to blend essential oils into products providing substances that will enhance your life.

Buying all the essential oils at the beginning of your essential oil adventure may not be cost effective. Research and experiment with blends of some of the more popular oils until you feel secure enough to branch out.

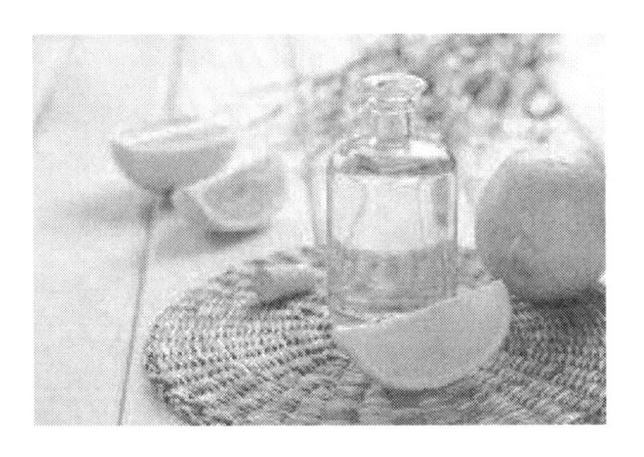

Lemon Essential Oil

Essential Oils to Keep on Hand for Recipes

Keep lemon essential oil on hand and replace it often. It is great for cleaning and degreasing. If you have something sticky on your hand, put a drop of lemon essential oil and rub it off. Add a few drops to your dishwater to help cut grease on dishes.

Lemon essential oil a great deodorizer. Stinky refrigerator? Add a few drops of lemon essential oil to a cup of baking soda. Just place it on the shelf in your refrigerator and it will absorb odors.

Mix one cup of water and one cup of vinegar in a spray bottle. Add 10 drops of lemon essential oil and use as a deodorizing spray.

Lavender is a must-have for any essential oil enthusiast. Lavender essential oil sooths the nerves and takes care of your skin. It induces peaceful sleep without the side effects of sleep aids and is great in many natural beauty recipes.

Personal Care Recipes

Lip Balm
2 tablespoons of calendula petals
2 tablespoons of marshmallow root
3 tablespoons of beeswax
½ cup of coconut oil
5 drops of peppermint essential oil
5 drops of lavender essential oil

Melt coconut oil on low heat and add herbs. Sit mixture for five minutes on low heat then transfer to warm oven.

Let the herbs steep in the oven for at least four hours. Strain the herbs from the oil and place it on the stove top on low heat.

Add the wax and let it melt.

Add the lavender and peppermint essential oils. If the aroma is not as strong as you like, add more drops of essential oil.

Pour into clean dry containers. Let it set up and use it as an awesome lip balm.

Tee tree oil is a great antimicrobial oil. It is a germ killer and can be added to cleaning sprays to kill germs. There are not harmful side effects with Tea tree oil and you can rest assured that your home is as germ-free with Tea tree essential oil as with large doses of chlorine bleach.

You can use tea tree essential oils in shampoo and conditioner recipes. Throw together this very simple shampoo recipe. It is a guarantee that there are no waxy or damaging additives in this recipe.

Shampoo

1 Tablespoon baking soda.
1 Cup of Water
Several drops of tea tree essential oil. Shake up until completely mixed and rinse well.
Conditioner (always use after shampooing)
1 Tablespoon apple cider vinegar – raw
1 Cup of water

Several drops of tea tree essential oil. Shake up and completely mix. Use in a squirt bottle. Apply, rinse.

Eucalyptus essential oil is a great addition to cleaning recipes. When mopping the floor add a couple squirts of castile soap and ten drops of eucalyptus essential oil to mop water. Use water and eucalyptus oil in a spray bottle to clean hardwood floors.

Keep Eucalyptus essential oils around to diffuse in the air when there are respiratory issues in your family. You can also add a couple of drops to a tablespoon of coconut oil to massage on your chest when you are having trouble breathing.

Peppermint is another essential oil that you need to keep on hand. It is antibacterial and analgesic plus soothes pain.

Peppermint is anti-inflammatory and great to use in the summer when you are hot and sweaty.

Cooling Off

Mix three drops of peppermint essential oil with one tablespoon of coconut oil. Apply to the back of your neck. You can also use this same mixture as a sore muscle rub.

Insect Repellents

55 drops of lemon eucalyptus. This is a good natural substitution for DEET. Do not use on children under three.
15 drops of cedar wood
15 drops of lavender
15 drops of rosemary

Add the essential liquids to a carrier and mix in a spray bottle. Shake well before using. You may need to reapply this bug repellent every few hours for maximum effect.

Other oils that have wonderful bug repelling properties include citronella, eucalyptus, tea tree, peppermint, cypress, rose geranium, bergamot and lemon.

Ant Repellent

Get rid of those pesky ants that love to trail along your kitchen floor and climb up to the countertops. Place a few drops of peppermint essential oil on a cotton ball and place where ants are crawling. Works well but can deplete your peppermint essential oil supply quickly.

Sunscreens

Use a carrier oil like coconut oil, shea butter, jojoba oil, sunflower or sesame oil. These oils are absorbed into the skin and provide natural sun protection. Add to your carrier oils eucalyptus and lavender essential oil. Eucalyptus has a low natural SPF and lavender will soothe your skin. Do not use citrus essential oils in sunscreens. They may increase sensitivity to sunlight.

1 oz. coconut oil

0.8 oz. shea butter

0.1oz. jojoba, sesame or sunflower oil

oz. Vitamin E oil

30 drops essential oils. Use 15 lavender, 10 eucalyptus, and 5 peppermint oil

Zinc oxide powder. Just bit for 2 oz. of lotion.

Add coconut oil, shea butter and jojoba/sesame/sunflower oils to a double boiler. Heat gently until shea butter melts. Remove from the double boiler and allow to cool. Add zinc oxide, vitamin E oil and essential oils. Combine well. Store in a dark jar in the refrigerator. Apply liberally to skin and reapply as needed. This preparation will keep for six months, however if you are out in the sun keep it in a cooler.

Sinus Infections

Sinusitis is an inflammation of the sinuses and can be caused by a virus, fungus or bacteria. When sinus openings become blocked from inflamed tissues or mucus build-up they can become infected. Antibiotics from your doctor are great, but essential oils and natural remedies are better.

There are a number of essential oils that have antimicrobial properties. These oils are very powerful in treating bacterial, viral and fungal infections. Use peppermint oil or eucalyptus in a humidifier to open up nasal passageways. Apply peppermint essential oil to the bridge of your nose. Dilute peppermint essential oil in a tablespoon of carrier oil. You can also put frankincense essential oil on your nose to clear up stuffiness.

Use a Neti pot to clear up a sinus infection. Irrigate using a saline solution with a drop of frankincense, rosemary and eucalyptus essential oil. Irrigate your nasal passages.

Massage Oil Recipes

Massage is the most well-known use of essential oils. You can make your own blends that help with different types of ailments.
Massage for Sore Muscles

2 drops of ginger
4 drops of cinnamon
3 drops of cajuput

3 drops of chamomile
15 ml of carrier oil
Mix with a good carrier and use as you would nay massage oils.
Work into muscles.
Massage for Fatigue Relief
6 drops of grapefruit
5 drops of palmarosa
4 drops of thyme
15 ml of carrier oil.

Shake well and use as needed. Take this to your massage therapist and introduce them to a new blend.

Calming Massage

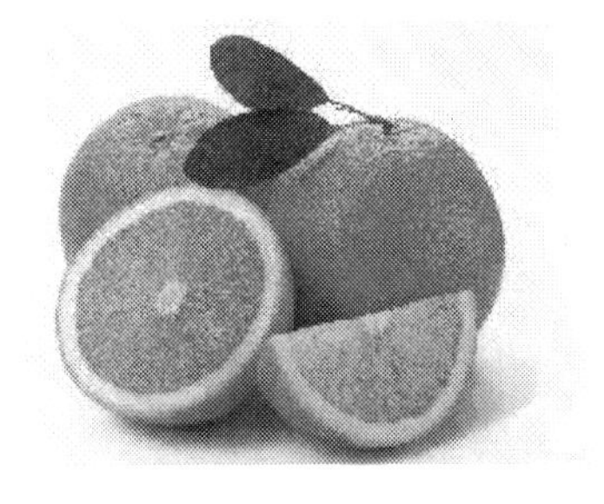

6 drops of petitgrain

5 drops of orange

4 drops of neroli

15 ml of carrier oil.

Blend well and massage into shoulders and back.

Inhaling Recipes

Perfumes and inhaling essential oils can enhance a good mood, chase away a bad day, relax you and bring you energy. You can feel glamorous, confident, exotic, or simply happy.

Confidence Spray

Two drops of basil

3 drops of bergamot

drop coriander

4 drops petitgrain

Add to a carrier oil or distilled water and mix in a spray bottle.

Self-esteem Spray

Two drops of ginger

Three drops of myrtle

Four drops of rosemary

Three drops of verbena

Add to a carrier oil or distilled water and mix in a spray bottle.

Calm Nerves

Four drops jasmine

Two drops lemon

One drop of patchouli

Add to a carrier oil or distilled water and mix in a spray bottle.

Stomach upset in a foreign country or at home can be helped with essential oils. Stay well-hydrated and add lemon essential oil to bottled water.

Five drops of lavender, geranium or ginger

One tablespoon of vegetable oil

Mix together with a carrier oil and massage over your stomach area.

Have a warm bath after applying this mixture.

Seek medical attention if your stomach ache worsens or you have diarrhea.

Relax & Rejuvenate

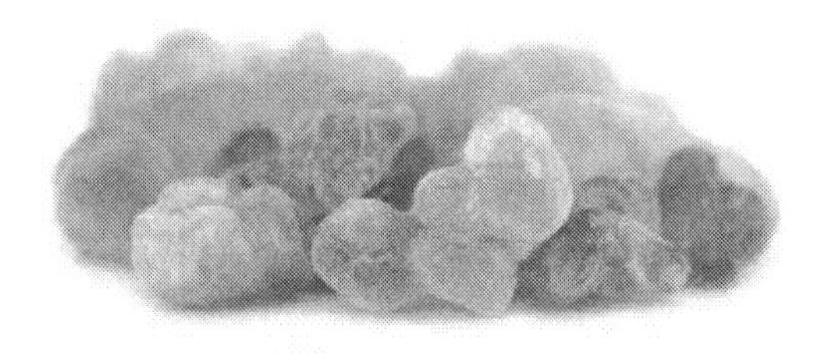

6 drops of wintergreen

6 drops of Lavender

drops of Peppermint

drops of frankincense

2 drops of basil

2 drops of rosemary

Mix together in a carrier oil and store in a dark, tightly lidded bottle.

If you are longing to be joyful, this essential oil recipe will bring you a feeling of happiness.

8 drops of lemon

drops of Melissa

4 drops of ylang-ylang

4 drops of sandalwood

Mix with a carrier oil like coconut or avocado. Store in a dark glass bottle and use as a very nice massage oil or drop 20 drops into a warm bath.

According to aromatherapists, essential oils bring synergy to the body. Synergy is the collaboration of elements that, when pooled together, produce a total outcome that is greater than the sum of the distinct elements, or contributions.

Chapter 8

Summary

"Essential oils embody the regenerating, oxygenating, and immune-strengthening properties of plants."

—Modern Essentials

Take charge of your health, be natural, and live green. Science is becoming more aware that essential oils, used thousands of years ago, do have a place in contemporary life. Medical communities are still somewhat skeptical that essential oils can be used in sufficient quantities to have any real curing power. Yet, it is proven that essential oils can move through the skin into the bloodstream quickly and with remarkable calming, stimulating or healing properties. The essence crosses the brain-blood barrier and move to all areas of the brain to decrease stress, increase stimulation, and provide emotional feelings of well-being.

Essential oils may not be able to cure diseases, but they do provide physical and emotional support that enhances the body's ability to fight diseases. Essential oils have also been known to delay the onset of disease symptoms.

Aromatherapy is the alternative medicine that sprang up because of essential oils. Aromatherapy brings in the therapeutic use of essential oils for improvement of physical, emotional and spiritual well-being.

Essential oils are volatile substances extracted from aromatic plant material by steam distillation or mechanical expression. There are a large array of chemical components that make up essential oils and these chemical components of are scientifically categorized as esters, terpenes, aldehydes, ketones, alcohols, phenols and oxides. Different essential oils contain varying amounts of these compounds and these are what make essential oils unique.

Companies

There are so many essential oils companies, it becomes confusing to know who is best to purchase your pure essential oils from. Distillers of essential oils caution beginners about purchasing oils that are not therapeutic-grade. Some excellent pointers for finding the best therapeutic essential oils include looking for companies that offer:

- Experience
- Purity
- Plants grown in indigenous locations
- Organic when possible
- Company that does not use pesticides, herbicides or harmful chemicals
- Reasonable shipping prices
- Reasonable pricing
- No solvents used in distillation
- No artificial oils sold in their line or products
- No adulterating, which mean no heating, blending, or additional distillation of oils
- Sourced from small farms
- They do not over recommend any of their oils, but educate the buyer on the properties and blends of essential oils.
- Find a company with a customer service department that is knowledgeable, friendly and helpful.

Ways to Use

A quick review of how you can use essential oils most effectively are:

- Bathing. Using essential oils in the bathtub is one of the easiest ways to benefit from the healing properties of essential oils.
- Room spray or potpourri will keep you from adding toxins to your home with commercial air fresheners.
- Sit down and soak your feet. Essential oils provide a special treat when added to a foot bath.
- Homemade body scrubs are the perfect way to exfoliate dry skin. Use a basic sugar or salt scrub recipe and add your favorite essential oil.
- Home cleaning needs essential oils with their antibacterial and anti-fungal properties. Add to homemade cleaners for a boost in benefits. Clean your toilets using essential oil, add them to detergents or fabric softeners.
- Use essential oils as skin moisturizers. Add a few drops of essential oil to a non-greasy moisturizing spray and have a light and soothing body spritz available.
- Facial cleansers with essential oils will provide you with astringent, anti-inflammatory and antibacterial properties.

- Bug repellents are very effective in keeping you and your family from being bitten.

- Massage oil is the most popular use of essential oils. All you need is a light carrier oil and three to five drops of an essential oil or blend.

- Oral hygiene can be augmented by essential oils. Just add a few drops of peppermint to your homemade toothpaste recipe and give the toothpaste companies a run for their money.

Different essential oils can be blended together to achieve a specific health benefit. When blended, the respective powers of the oils do not change, but are enhanced. Blend essential oils and experiment, but if you have a recipe, and you are an essential oil beginner, follow the recipe until you are familiar with the scents and traits of the most used essential oils.

When you have selected an essential oil you like, add it to base products and enhance your favorite health and beauty items. You can dilute essential oils simply by adding them to unscented bath oils, lotions, massage lotions and shower gels.

Follow these dilution suggestions and you will have a good start for using essential oils:

- Massage – five drops of essential oil per teaspoon of base oil

- Inhalation – one to two drops in boiling water

- Bath – eight to ten drops in bath water
- Sauna – two drops to 2 ½ cups of water
- Facials – two to three drops in a base
- Cleanser – 20 drops in four ounces of base product
- Chest Rub – 10-20 drops to one o of carrier oil
- Laundry – 10-20 drops per load

Combine essential oils with carrier oils that are pure. Almond oil, jojoba oil, olive oil, grapeseed oil, avocado oil and coconut oil are perfect carriers for your essential oils. Keep a stock of any of these oils on hand and add your favorite essential oils to them.

Use your essential blends or single oils in laundry detergent, salt scrub for your skin, refresh your furniture, for mouthwash, and lavender oil with aloe vera gel for burns. Add it to vinegar for laundry softeners and you can use lavender essential oil in enemas.

Aromatherapy and essential oils are based on smell. Aromatherapy uses the oils extracted from flowers, leaves, roots, seeds, fruit and bark for special blends that work in harmony the body to provide a sense of well-being. Essential oils are natural. What they possess is almost impossible to reproduce outside of nature. For a healing and balanced life, use pure essential oils and find yourself one with nature.

References

Ajowan Oil. (n.d.). Retrieved March 5, 2015, from http://www.kanta-group.com/ajowan-oil.htm

Aromatherapy (Essential Oils Therapy) – Topic Overview. (2015). Retrieved March 5, 2015, from webmd.com

Banks, J. S. (2013, September 18). 5 essential oils that heal. Retrieved March 5, 2015, from http://www.foxnews.com/health/2013/09/18/5-essential-oils-that-heal/

Essential Oil First Aid Kit–Essential Oils Pedia. (2013, August 05). Retrieved March 5, 2015, from http://www.essentialoilspedia.com/essential-oil-first-aid-kit/

Essential Oils for Dogs. (n.d.). Retrieved March 5, 2015, from http://www.weedemandreap.com/essential-oils-dogs/

Essential Oils. (n.d.). Retrieved March 5, 2015, from https://www.organicfacts.net/health-benefits/essential-oils

Healing Power of Lavender Oil. (n.d.). Retrieved March 5, 2015, from http://www.theconfidentmom.com/09/essential-oils/healing-cuts-burns-and-wounds-with-lavender-oil/

Homemade Bug Spray Recipes That Work! (2011, June 10). Retrieved March 5, 2015, from http://wellnessmama.com/2565/homemade-bug-spray/

Inhabitat | Design For a Better World! (n.d.). Retrieved March 5, 2015, from http://inhabitat.com/

Natural Wound Healing Made Easy With Essential Oils. (n.d.). Retrieved March 5, 2015, from http://www.experience-essential-oils.com/natural-wound-healing.html

The Essential Oil Company – Your Essential Oils Source. (n.d.). Retrieved March 5, 2015, from http://www.essentialoi.com

Well+Good. (n.d.). Retrieved March 5, 2015, from http://wellandgood.com

What Is an Essential Oil? (n.d.). Retrieved from http://www.doterra.com/sgen/essentialDefininitn.php

Conclusion

Thank you again for downloading this book!

I hope this book was able to help you to get excited about essential oils.

The next step is to look for more books on essential oils and natural living.

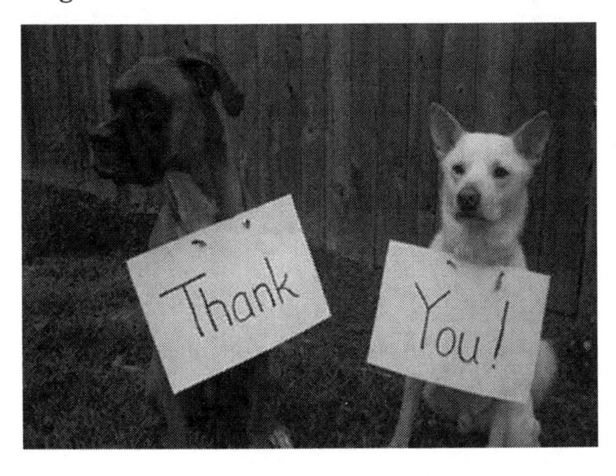

Finally, if you enjoyed this book, then I'd like to ask you for a favor, would you be kind enough to leave a review for this book on Amazon? It'd be greatly appreciated!

Click here to leave a review for this book on Amazon!

Thank you!

Joy Louis

About Author Joy Louis:

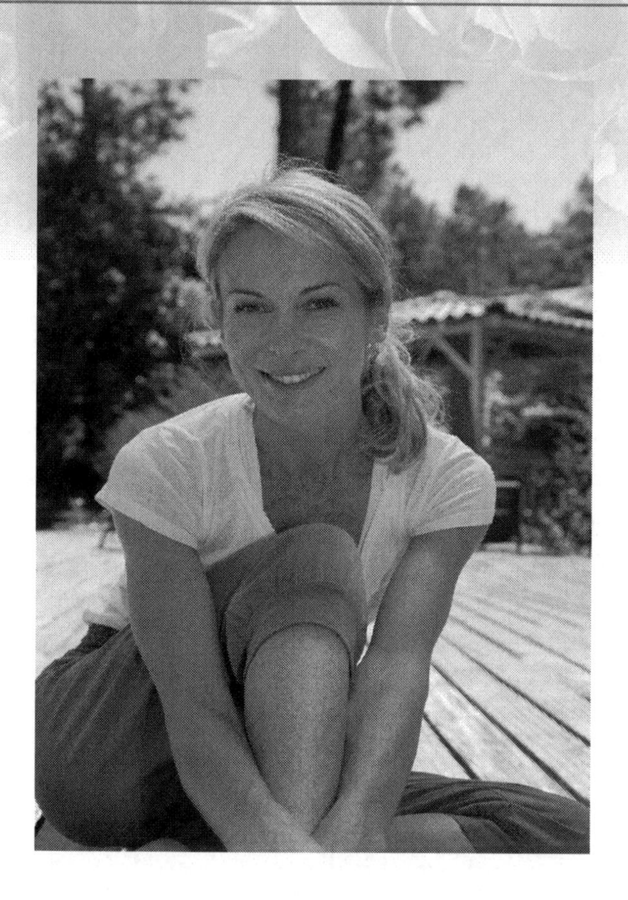

Hello there! I'm Joy Louis, a lifelong learner, student and seeker of knowledge in natural health and alternative medicine. My life is full of abundance My current residence is in Los Angeles, CA where me and my loving husband share a beautiful life together. Let's connect on Facebook here -> https://www.facebook.com/JoyLouisBooks

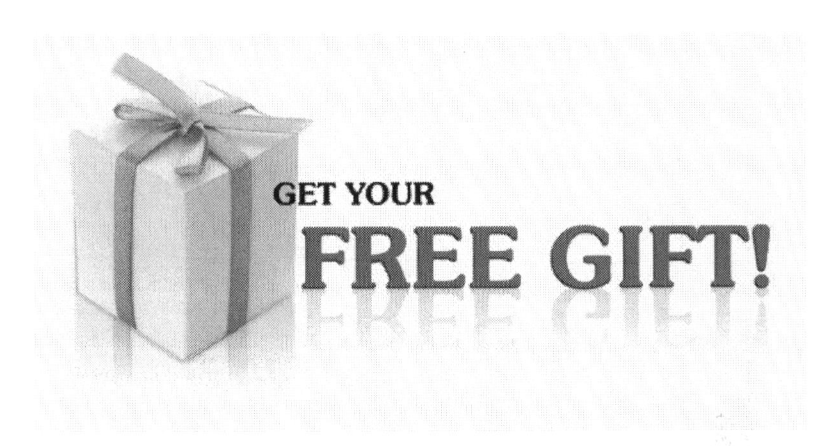

WAIT! – DO YOU LIKE FREE BOOKS?

My **FREE Gift** to You!! As a way to say **Thank You** for downloading my book, I'd like to offer you more **FREE BOOKS!** Each time we release a NEW book, we offer it first to a small number of people as a test–drive. Because of your commitment here in downloading my book, I'd love for you to be a part of this group. You can join easily here→ **http://joylouisbooks.com/**

Do You Enjoy **FREE BOOKS**? Do you like books that are Life Changing, Inspirational, Motivational and Informative? We **LOVE** sharing **FREE BOOKS** with people like you. It's easy to join just by clicking here→ **http://joylouisbooks.com/**

Made in the USA
San Bernardino, CA
20 December 2015